Day Surgery for Nurses

Day Surgery for Nurses

Edited by
Louise Markanday

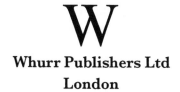

Whurr Publishers Ltd
London

© 1997 Whurr Publishers Ltd
First published 1997 by
Whurr Publishers Ltd
19b Compton Terrace, London N1 2UN, England

British Library Cataloguing in Publication Data
A catalogue record for this book is available from the
British Library.

ISBN 1 86156 038 9

Printed and bound in the UK by Athenaeum Press Ltd,
Gateshead, Tyne & Wear

Contents

Contributors

Gina Behar-Spicer, RGN, DPSN
Sister, Day Surgical Unit, Southlands Hospital, Shoreham-by-Sea

Sharon Bole, RGN, RSCN
Paediatric Lead Nurse, Day Surgery Unit, Kingston Hospital

Debra Green, RDN, RCNT, MMEd formerly Senior Lecturer
(Day Surgery), Faculty of Healthcare Sciences, Kingston University
and St George's Medical School

Basia Howard-Harwood, RN Dip, BSc(Hons) formerly Staff
Nurse, Day Surgical Unit, Southlands Hospital, Shoreham-by-Sea

Louise Markanday, RGN Lecturer/Practitioner in Day Surgery
Nursing, Southlands Hospital, Shoreham-by-Sea and the University
of Brighton

Rosemary Mitchell, RGN Senior Staff Nurse (Anaesthetics), Day
Surgical Unit, Southlands Hospital, Shoreham-by-Sea

Jacqui Rollason, SRN Staff Nurse, Day Surgery Unit, Kingston
Hospital

Sarah Williams, RGN, Dip.HE (Health Studies) formerly Theatre Lead Nurse, Day Surgery Unit, Kingston Hospital

Dawn Wotton, RGN, DPSN Senior Sister, Day Surgery Unit, Kingston Hospital

Acknowledgements

Chapter 3

The authors are grateful to Dr NG Lavies, Consultant Anaesthetist at Worthing and Southlands Hospital NHS Trust, for his help in the laborious task of reading through the chapter, tirelessly correcting inaccuracies; Dr D Uncles, Consultant Anaesthetist, Worthing and Southlands Hospital NHS Trust, for proofreading and giving us ideas; Charlotte Stoneham, Senior Pharmacist, Southlands Hospital, for checking drug actions and side effects throughout the chapter; our colleagues on the Day Surgical Unit at Southlands Hospital for putting up with us being constantly engrossed in the preparation of this chapter; and our children, Sam, Sophie, Hannah, Nathan and Naomi, who throughout the writing of this chapter were virtually ignored by their respective mothers.

Chapter 6

The author would like to thank several individuals for their support and guidance: Maire Woolven, Anthea Cross, Margaret Norris and Sue Marling for developing my interest in nursing and day surgery; Louise Markanday for her unending words of encouragement and never fading support in writing this chapter; and my husband, Mark, and my parents.

Chapter 1
A brief history and the development of day surgery

Louise Markanday

Introduction

Day-case surgery is defined by the *Concise Oxford Medical Dictionary* (1994, p. 168) as 'surgical procedures that can be performed in a single day, without the need to admit the patient for an overnight stay in hospital ...'. It is this definition that is understood by the term 'day surgery' in the UK. However, in the USA the term 'ambulatory surgery' is more commonly used, and this often means a post-operative stay of up to 23 hours and 59 minutes.

This short chapter is intended to give the reader a background knowledge of the history and development of day surgery. It examines changes in attitudes towards health care and looks briefly at the history of surgery and nursing from ancient times to the present. It also examines the social factors that once made day surgery undesirable, and explores the technological and pharmacological advances made during the past 150 years. The earliest documented examples of day surgery are presented.

An attempt is also made to predict likely developments in day surgery during the next 10 years, and the nurse's role in taking day surgery into the next century is explored.

A brief history of day surgery

At first glance, the history of day surgery may appear to be a relatively short one, as generally, day surgery has been embraced in both the UK and USA only during the last 50 years or so. However, it is worth considering what our ancient relatives achieved in the way of surgery and the social and economic changes that combined to make day surgery both possible and desirable.

1

It could be argued that the concept of day surgery is nothing new. There is evidence to suggest that the ancient Egyptians, Greeks and Romans all performed day surgery of some kind (Singer, 1993). As there is little or no mention of hospitals, it is to be assumed that the patient recovered from surgery in his or her own home.

Surgery and medicine

Translations from papyrus scrolls indicate that the Egyptians were probably at the forefront of developments in surgery and had 'specialists' for different parts of the body. The translations indicate that the Egyptians diagnosed and followed a rational methodology in performing lithotomies, castration, amputations, eye operations, and wound cleansing and closure (Singer, 1993). Homer alludes to the drugs of Egypt.

The era of scientific medicine began with Hippocrates, who demanded high moral and ethical standards from physicians, and asserted that disease was not due to demons but to natural causes. The Hippocratic oath bears his name and is still accepted to this day. Homer's *Iliad* (written about 1200–1000 BC) makes many references to the treatment of complex battle wounds, and Hippocrates wrote on diverse medical problems from the treatment of club foot to head injuries (Singer, 1993). Hippocrates also appears to have been aware of nursing skills, such as bandaging and bathing, though he did not leave any actual writings on nursing.

Apart from midwives, none of the ancient civilisations appear to have had nurses. Patients were presumably nursed by their relatives or slaves. In the event of a Roman slave becoming ill, he or she was cast into the temple at the mercy of the gods. Claudius (d. 54 AD) decreed that if slaves recovered from their illnesses, then they could claim their freedom. One wonders just how many did recover when it is remembered that there were no antibiotics and, presumably, they were exposed to the elements! The Romans did not have public hospitals, but did have public doctors who would attend to the poor free of charge in the provinces.

Illness and disease were frequently attributed to the anger of the gods and goddesses, but as a causal relationship between disaster and physical phenomena was observed, the Greeks began to question these beliefs and the consequent rise of scholarship and science caused a crisis in these religious doctrines. Christianity, however, appealed to the philosophers as a rational system of thought, and was based on service to the poor, the humble and one's neighbours. However, its attitude to life was ambivalent, in that this life had to be endured with patience and suffering in order to ensure everlasting life.

After the spread of Christianity, records of hospitals and medicine become scarce and the medical advances of the early Greeks were discounted because of their Pagan origins (Schneck, 1984); mysticism, witchcraft and demonology took their place.

During the Middle Ages the care of the sick and wounded fell mainly to the monasteries, and these infirmaries used medicinal herbs and plants. Hospitals were founded by religious orders along the routes of the crusades, such as the Knights of St John. St Bartholomew's Hospital in London is an example of an early religious hospital.

War, through necessity, has played and continues to play a large part in the development of surgery (Rutkow, 1993; Gordon, 1993). One has only to consider the advances made in plastic surgery during the Second World War to support this view. At the beginning of the nineteenth century a rather disorganised system of medical care was in operation, and patients trusted doctors on the basis of how the physician behaved more than because of any success he might have had. Much of the knowledge accrued by doctors was still based on the ancient Greek and Roman writings. High prestige was attached to physicians, and many of the bloodcurdling remedies frequently employed were accepted by patients because of the high status enjoyed by doctors (Dingwall, Rafferty & Webster, 1988). At this time hospitals were still few and far between and any nursing required by patients was performed by servants in the richer classes and by relatives in the poorer ones. The nurses employed in what hospitals there were, were untrained and often of dubious character.

During the past 200 years major advancements have been made in medicine and surgery. In 1846 William Thomas Morton demonstrated ether anaesthesia in Massachusetts, USA (Smith & White, 1994). Despite its obvious importance, the concept of anaesthesia was slow to progress. In 1865 Lord Lister devised antisepsis in surgery (Gordon, 1993), with his steam-driven carbolic-spray, and microbes were discovered by Pasteur at the end of the nineteenth century. In 1895 X-rays were discovered accidentally by Rontgen, and in 1898 Pierre and Marie Curie discovered radium. All these discoveries have contributed to what we know today as medicine and surgery.

Nursing

As medicine progressed and science advanced, a need for nurses with the knowledge to care for patients within hospitals was recognised. In 1860 the Nightingale School of Nursing at St Thomas's Hospital was established by Florence Nightingale, and towards the end of the century other establishments for the training of young women to become nurses were opened in major hospitals throughout the country. The Nightingale model for nurse training was copied throughout the civilised world and her *Notes on Nursing* became medical classics. 'Nightingale nurses' were in great demand and the movement quickly made its way to the USA (Rutkow, 1993).

Young women were normally recruited from the upper or middle classes and they were often required to fund themselves through their training. The hours on duty were long, and time off limited. The pay was also poor. In 1901 in London, a nurse received a salary of £26 10s (£26.50) at a time when a female certified teacher was paid £80. However, a nurse could expect to have her uniform provided and often received some board and lodging.

Once training for nurses had been widely introduced, there existed a varied group of people practising nursing. Some were young women who had received excellent instruction; others servant girls who had had only the rudiments of training, if any at all. There was no control over the standard of training a probationer nurse would receive, so the fact that a nurse was trained did not automatically imply a certain standard of expertise.

In 1916 the College of Nursing Ltd was established with the aims of promoting education and training of nurses and to lobby parliament continually for official recognition of nurses. This was later to be granted a Royal charter.

As the suffragette movement gained momentum at the turn of the century, nurses (all female) felt that they were gaining ground. In 1919 the Nurses Registration Act was finally passed and only those nurses admitted to the national register of nurses were entitled to call themselves 'nurse'. To be admitted to the register, a period of training in an approved school had to have been completed. The first State examination was held in 1922, and from then on admittance to the register was only by successful completion of this examination.

Since this major milestone in the history of the profession many changes have taken place. However, the fundamental ideals of the original act remain, and the visions of the early nursing pioneers have materialised and continue to be built upon.

The development of day surgery

At the beginning of the twentieth century it was usual for patients to remain in hospital after surgery or when ill. Sanatoriums for the treatment of infectious and largely incurable diseases, such as tuberculosis, were widespread. The trend was to keep people in hospital for their own good; the only reference to day surgery appears to be the work of Nicoll in the early 1900s. He reported performing surgery on 8,988 children as day cases over a 10-year period (Smith & White, 1994) at the Glasgow Royal Hospital for Sick Children.

The lack of day surgery can, perhaps, be attributed to the poor social conditions of the time. Housing for the working classes was poor and many homes had neither running water nor electricity. In fact, one can suppose that the majority of the population would not have met the criteria for day surgery which are deemed so essential nowadays. Prolonged rest was also considered vital for successful recovery either from surgery or from illness, and hospital was thought to be the best place for patients by both the nursing and medical professions. The anaesthetics then in use caused considerable post-operative nausea and vomiting; the importance of good hygiene was not as widely understood as nowadays and, without antibiotics, wound infection was a very real concern which could, and often did, prove fatal. The working population was largely poorly educated and knew little, if anything, about the workings of their own bodies. At the turn of the century illiteracy was common.

The concept of day surgery appears to have first taken hold in the USA. Phippen (1992) recalls undergoing tonsillectomy at the doctors' surgery in 1952 in the USA. He recovered from the anaesthesia at home. As a child of seven, he recalls the feeling of security at being able to return home with his parents. However, in the UK today, tonsillectomy is still often not performed as a day case!

In the USA it was mainly the insurance companies who pushed for the growth of day surgery. Indeed, for some procedures they would only reimburse the patient if the surgery had been performed as a day case, as costs were reduced by not keeping the patient in hospital.

Since the inception of the National Health Service in the UK in 1947, free health care has been available for all, and only those who choose it have private treatment. As a consequence, there was not the same incentive for day surgery to develop on this side of the Atlantic. However, as the cost of health care has increased dramatically in the 50 years since the formation of the NHS (due to massive technological advances and knowledge), the desire and need for cheaper ways of delivering care have increased.

Before the 1980s the provision of day surgery was sporadic. Farquson reported successfully performing day-case inguinal hernia repairs in 1955, and during the 1960s and 1970s day surgery was performed in Aberdeen, Edinburgh, London, Birmingham, Kingston and Cambridge.

It was in the late 1980s that day surgery really began to develop an identity of its own in the UK. The cost of health care was becoming an ever bigger issue and this drove many hospitals to establish day-care services. The Royal College of Surgeons published its *Guidelines for Day Case Surgery* in 1985, and stated that 50 per cent of all surgical cases need not remain in hospital overnight. This report was considered a breakthrough, and by the early 1990s most hospitals had a dedicated day surgical unit (DSU) or treated many surgical cases on a day-stay basis. However, as Ghosh (1996) found in his audit of day surgery provision in the UK, there remains a wide regional variation in the way in which day surgery is provided.

The multidisciplinary British Association of Day Surgery was formed in 1989 to promote quality day surgery, encourage research and to provide meetings for the sharing of innovations and ideas.

Social conditions have also improved enough to allow day surgery to be possible. It is rare for somebody to live in a house without plumbing, electricity or access to a telephone. The population is better educated and many have considerable knowledge of their body from school, through reading magazine articles and from watching television documentaries. Illiteracy is not as common as it once was.

Surgical techniques and the quality of anaesthesia have also played their part in the development of day surgery. Minimally invasive surgery (MIS) or 'keyhole surgery' has become more commonplace over the last decade and this technique undoubtedly is suitable for day surgery. Post-operative pain is reduced as the actual procedure is not as invasive as conventional methods, and because the wound is only tiny, the risk of infection is reduced. Many people are able to return to work far sooner after MIS than after conventional surgery.

New anaesthetic-inducing drugs that do not cause a hangover effect were introduced during the 1980s. As a result, patients do not suffer the prolonged after-effects of anaesthesia associated with older, traditional drugs. The Laryngeal Mask Airway (LMA) was also invented, reducing the need for intubation and so creating a more pleasant anaesthetic for the patient. More information on all these issues is given later in the book.

The NHS management executive (Ghosh, 1996) requests that two thirds of all elective surgery should be carried out as day cases by 1997. This is a high figure to achieve, especially when it is remembered that the population of the UK is getting older. The next section examines the implications of such dictates and looks at the influence of professionals in achieving these targets.

Changes in attitude by the caring professions

Over the past 20 years or so the rights of the patient have been recognised by both the nursing and medical professions. The air of conspiracy which was common in medical circles during the 1950s has largely disappeared. Patients feel more able to question the decisions of professionals and are usually given a say in the kind of treatment they will receive. Day surgery fits neatly into this philosophy. For day surgery to be successful the patient must take responsibility for his own wellbeing and welfare. Studies have shown that this new concept has, in general, been favourably received by patients (Buttery et al., 1993; Lyall, 1995).

The medical profession has been slower to accept the concept of day surgery. Some anaesthetists find the idea of sending a patient home two or three hours after receiving a general anaesthetic difficult to comprehend and consequently err on the side of caution. Surgeons in the UK do not seem to enjoy the same ego satisfaction or status from day surgery (Kark, 1996) as their colleagues in the USA. Many simply prefer to perform more complicated major surgery and find the minor surgery carried out in DSUs tedious and monotonous. For a DSU to be successful, it needs to have strong leadership from a senior clinician and senior nurse who are both motivated and dedicated to the ideal of day surgery. There is, however, evidence that matters are improving all the time and that the incidence of day surgery is increasing nationally (Kark, 1996).

In recent years nurses have embraced the concept of an holistic approach to care, which entails caring for the entire person and not just one physical component. As a consequence, their assessment and information-giving skills have improved and nurse training now reflects this. Recent major changes to nurses' training have altered the emphasis of the care of the patient to community care and study of the well person. This has resulted in the inclusion of day surgery, with its emphasis on self-care and recovery in the home, in the nursing students' syllabus and means day surgery is seen as a progressive specialty by the profession as a whole.

The public perception of day care

Day surgery has been viewed with a certain amount of suspicion by some members of the public, while others have welcomed the chance to have surgery without a stay in hospital. Many people still fear hospitals, and even those who have no fear do not particularly like the experience of a hospital stay. However, the public have very real fears about day surgery as well. Pain after surgery is a common fear, and the anxiety of what to do if something goes wrong is experienced by both patients and carers. Education and information-giving is vital for day surgery to be successful and all these issues are covered in depth in subsequent chapters.

On the positive side, the idea of being able to attend a DSU and be home after surgery within a matter of hours is appealing to both adults and children. Most people prefer to recover in their own bed and surroundings, and children benefit from not being separated from their parents and siblings. Experience suggests that as long as certain rules are followed by the professionals, most patients prefer the day surgery experience to a lengthy hospital stay.

The future

It is always difficult to predict future trends, but it does seem that day surgery is here to stay. Most UK hospitals offer day surgery in one form or another; in the USA day surgery is widespread and in Australia it is also prolific. The rest of Europe is catching up, and in developing countries day surgery is often the only kind of surgery on offer.

It is likely that all minor and intermediate surgery will be performed on a day-stay basis within the next 30 years and the only patients in hospital will be those who require major surgery or who are seriously ill. We have already seen an increase in community care in the past 10 years and it seems logical to assume that this trend will continue. Advancements in anaesthesic techniques will enable access to day surgery to those excluded at the moment. Surgical techniques will improve and MIS will develop further so enabling easier day surgery.

There may be 'drop-in' DSUs where patients may refer themselves and arrange surgery around their own work and family commitments. These may be run by the NHS or private consortia. As money becomes more scarce within the NHS certain surgical interventions may be funded only as long as they are carried out as a day case.

It is exciting to think that day surgery will continue to develop at a rapid pace and that a new nursing specialty will emerge. However, there will always be some patients who do not recover sufficiently from their surgery for discharge and provision must always be made for these individuals. There will also be those for whom day surgery will never be a safe option because of existing disease or social conditions. In the planning of future DSUs these people must not be overlooked. Hospital hotels are a good alternative to a hospital stay where medical or nursing intervention is not required. In their quest for more day surgery, it is to be hoped that politicians do not forget those who cannot have day surgery and that these people are not be penalised.

Many of the disadvantages of day surgery can be overcome through careful preparation and education, and by the middle of the next century it is likely that day surgery will be accepted by all and the idea of having to stay in hospital after surgery will seem as foreign to patients as day surgery appears to some today. Nurses must be at the forefront of these developments and ensure that their training and education keeps abreast of the continuing evolution of day surgery.

References

Buttery Y, Sissons J, Williams KN (1993) Patients' views one week after day surgery with general anaesthesia. Journal of One Day Surgery 3(1): 6–8.

Dingwall R, Rafferty AM, Webster C (1988) An Introduction to the Social History of Nursing. London: Routledge.

Ghosh S (1996) Is the development of UK day surgery good enough? Journal of One Day Surgery 5(4): 14–15.

Gordon R (1993) The Alarming History of Medicine. London: Sinclair-Stevenson.

Kark A (1996) Editorial. Day surgery specialisation. Journal of One Day Surgery 6(1): 1.

Lyall J (1995) Gains and pains. Health Service Journal 105(5440): 1–2.

Oxford Concise Medical Dictionary, 4th edn (1994) Oxford: Oxford University Press.

Phippen M (1992) Editorial. Ambulatory surgery in 1952. Seminars in Perioperative Nursing 1(4): iv–v.

Royal College of Surgeons (1985) Report of the Working Party on Guidelines for Day Case Surgery. London: Royal College of Surgeons.

Rutkow IM (1993) Surgery – An Illustrated History. St Louis: Mosby-Year Book.

Schneck LH (1984) Ambulatory surgery. AORN Journal 40(2): 248–250.

Singer HK (1993) Then and now: a historical development of ambulatory surgery. Journal of Post Anaesthesia Nursing 8(4): 276–279.

Smith I, White PF (1994) History and scope of day-case anaesthesia: past, present and future. In Whitwam JG (Ed) Day-Case Anaesthesia and Sedation. Oxford: Blackwell Scientific Publications.

Further reading

Abel-Smith B (1960) A History of the Nursing Profession. London: Heinemann.
Baly M (1973) Nursing and Social Change. London: William Heinemann Medical
    Books.
Maggs C (1983) The Origins of General Nursing. London: Croom Helm.

Chapter 2
Selection and pre-assessment of the day surgery patient

Louise Markanday

Introduction

For many patients requiring minor surgery a day stay is the preferred option. However, not all patients can safely have their surgery as a day case, either because they have a medical condition that can affect the outcome of a general anaesthetic, or because their home circumstances are not conducive to successful recovery from surgery and anaesthesia. Before accepting a patient for day surgery, it is the clinician's responsibility to ensure that the surgery required is suitable to be performed as a day case, that the patient has no medical condition likely to preclude day surgery and that his or her social situation is adequate.

Accurate assessment of the patient's fitness for anaesthesia is vital if day surgery is to be successful and uncomplicated. Nurses are well equipped to perform this role because they possess good communication skills and are traditionally perceived by the patient to be more approachable than doctors. Irvine et al. (1995, p. 5) said, 'In units where assessment is delegated to a nurse improvements have been identified by both consultants and nurses'.

This chapter aims to assist the nurse in setting up a pre-assessment clinic in his or her area and to work within the multidisciplinary team to ensure that patient safety is maintained. It examines the nurse's role in detail and attempts to explain why all day surgery patients

11

should be assessed prior to admission. It also explores the wider concept of pre-assessment against simple selection for suitability and medical screening, and explains the criteria for acceptance used by most day surgical units (DSUs).

The skills required by the nurse are described, and there is discussion on whether pre-assessment is necessary for the smooth running of a DSU, or an expensive, time-consuming luxury. The advantages and disadvantages for both patient and staff are examined. The chapter explores the use of a nursing framework and offers some ideas on documentation. There are also some suggestions on how nurses may be sufficiently educated and trained to fulfil this important role effectively.

The selection of patients for day surgery

The selection of patients is the identification of those patients who require surgery that may be performed on a day-stay basis. These patients must also be fit to have a general anaesthetic (GA). Doctors undertake the task of selection.

Accurate diagnosis is vital before the patient can be considered for day surgery. In its report *A Short Cut to Better Services*, the Audit Commission (1990) described 20 procedures, known as the 'basket of procedures', deemed suitable for day surgery. This list included such procedures as laparoscopy, excision of lumps and bumps, arthroscopy and other minor surgical procedures. Although many units now perform procedures outside this original list it is still considered absolutely essential that the surgery will last no longer than an hour and that the patient will not require prolonged hospital admission post-operatively. No complications during surgery should be anticipated and the expected level of pain afterwards should not be so high as to require admission to hospital for the administration of regular intramuscular or intravenous analgesia. The surgeon who first sees the patient in out-patients must take all these factors into account before deciding to admit the patient to the DSU. He or she should also consider the patient's fitness to receive a general anaesthetic as a day case following the American Society of Anesthesiologists morbidity classification (see Chapter 3 for details), and consideration must also be given to the patient's social circumstances. It is desirable that the surgeon who will be performing the surgery assesses the patient, as different surgeons are prepared to do different procedures as day surgery. The doctor should be of at least registrar grade to possess the necessary level of skill in assessment and accurate diagnosis required for the successful planning of day surgery.

The Association of Anaesthetists of Great Britain and Ireland (1994) has produced a booklet outlining its recommendations for day surgery. The largest section of this booklet is devoted to the subject of patient selection, a measure of the importance anaesthetists place on this process. In most hospitals, the ultimate decision as to whether a patient should receive a general anaesthetic is made by the anaesthetist and, therefore, the same applies within a day surgery setting. However, the demands on a modern anaesthetist in a large hospital are considerable and there may not be time for every anaesthetist to personally pre-assess his or her patient for day surgery. Therefore, in many cases, the anaesthetist has to rely on the skill of colleagues to accurately select patients for day surgery.

Guidelines on selection

Every DSU should lay down criteria for acceptance of patients, which are agreed by all parties regardless of who will be performing the actual assessment. Most units follow the recommendations of the Royal College of Surgeons (1992), which are:

1. The patient should be of physical status ASA I, normally healthy people, or II, those with minor systemic disease not interfering with normal activities, including medical conditions that are well controlled with therapy.
2. The patient must be able to have an adult with him or her for the first 24 hours after discharge, must have access to a telephone at home and must have someone to accompany them home.
3. The proposed surgery will not take longer than an hour and the after-care will not require intensive nursing.
4. The patient is willing to have his or her surgery performed as a day case.

If the above protocol is followed then the patient should have a safe and successful passage through day surgery. The patient can be safely discharged into the care of his or her family with community nurse or general practitioner (GP) support if necessary.

More information on why guidelines are so vital for day surgery anaesthesia is contained later in this chapter and in greater depth in Chapter 3.

The selection of patients for day surgery is a process that ensures that the patient fulfils the criteria for day surgery but does not meet any other needs, such as the giving of information to enable the patient to comply with instructions, pre-operative preparation, discharge planning, psychological support, counselling on the proposed surgery, and the giving of pre- and post-operative advice. Nurses are well suited and qualified to fulfil these needs and the next section explains how and why nurse pre-assessment should be adopted.

Pre-assessment by nurses

Pre-assessment is defined by Markanday and Platzer (1994, pp.38–42) as 'a pre-admission interview between nurse and patient in which the patient is assessed for his or her physical, psychological and social suitability to have their surgery performed as a day case. It is also a time during which the patient is psychologically prepared for the operation and given pre-operative instructions to follow and post-operative advice so that he or she can plan for their discharge.'

In DSUs where pre-assessment is undertaken by nurses, improvements in patient selection and preparation have been noted by both nursing and medical staff (Irvine et al., 1995) and prior to the introduction of pre-assessment many nurses felt that the social needs of the day surgery patient were largely ignored (Reynolds & Morgan, 1991).

In its *Guidelines for Day Case Surgery* the Royal College of Surgeons (1992) states that suitability should be assessed and recognises the important and invaluable role that nurses make in the pre-assessment of patients. When this process is in place, patients arrive for surgery fit for anaesthetic, avoiding the last minute cancellation of patients which wastes operating time. The number of patients requiring overnight admission after surgery is also reduced, which clearly has economic implications.

The requirements of the *Patients' Charter* (Department of Health, 1992) are also met through the pre-assessment of patients. It provides the opportunity to explain proposed treatment and identify a named nurse.

Nursing assessment skills

During the assessment process, information or data will be gathered by the nurse. These data may be based on personal observation (subjective) or may be physically measured data (e.g. vital sign observations), which are often referred to as objective data. It is often assumed that objective data are more accurate than subjective data, but there have been instances where it has been clearly demonstrated that both are of equal importance during the assessment process (Thomas, Wearing and Bennett, 1991).

A comprehensive assessment of an individual in any clinical setting must include the biological, psychological, social and spiritual aspects (Allcock, 1996), and any guidelines laid down to assist nurses in the role must encompass these. Both subjective and objective data must be collected on these issues.

Nursing students are taught assessment skills during their training. However, it can be argued that many do not understand the theory behind successful and useful assessment. The first step is data collection. This is the interview with the patient, where questions are asked to obtain information and responses to specified questions are recorded. The second step is the interpretation of collected data, and the third step is the use of the information to plan care.

Questions must be posed in a manner that is understood by the patient and in the language which he or she speaks. This is not only language in the sense of the mother tongue, but also by judging if he or she is able to understand medical and nursing terminology or jargon. Eye contact should be maintained and both nurse and patient should be able to sit comfortably and not be in a position where their conversation may be overheard by others. The interview can be classified as the collection of both subjective and objective data. Measurable information, such as blood pressure reading, is gathered, as well as verbal responses from the patient about his or her medical status. The nurse is also observing the patient and making assumptions based on that observation. The nurse should have the patient's notes and have familiarised her or himself with the patient's relevant past medical history before beginning the interview. The assessment process should begin even before the nurse and patient have had a chance to speak to one another. The nurse should look at the patient and note his or her general demeanour. Does he or she appear relaxed, or nervous and agitated? How does the patient respond to being called? Does he or she become flustered or remain calm, or is there an appearance of relief?

Nurses are ideally equipped to pre-assess patients for day surgery as they possess good communication skills and patients often feel more comfortable with a nurse than they do with a doctor. Nurses are perceived to be more approachable and of lower status than their medical colleagues, and patients will often confide in a nurse information which has been withheld from a doctor.

Organisation of pre-assessment

The method of pre-assessing patients varies considerably from unit to unit. Many units only pre-assess those patients who are to have a GA, as those who are to have their procedure performed under a local anaesthetic (LA) do not need to have medical screening for fitness for anaesthesia. However, as medical screening is only one component of pre-assessment, this policy does raise other issues for the latter group of patients, and these will be discussed later in the chapter.

In the ideal situation all patients should be pre-assessed, but most units find this to be practically impossible because of constraints on resources. Some units favour a separate clinic for the purpose of pre-assessment, which means that the assessing nurse can concentrate solely on the pre-assessment clinic and not be in competition with the demands of the DSU. Some units have a day surgery nurse who sits in on out-patient clinics to pre-assess the patient immediately after consultation with the doctor. The main disadvantage of this is that the nurse is removed from the DSU team, which may cause staffing problems. Another disadvantage is that the patient may not actually visit the unit and may, therefore, be anxious about where to go on the day of surgery. Whichever method is chosen, the vital element required is time, and the staffing budget must take pre-assessment into account when being set.

Ideally, the patient should be pre-assessed at the same time as the out-patient consultation. However, this poses difficulties for the unit as it means that patients turn up for pre-assessment without appointments, and as most units are extremely busy, this method is often viewed as impractical. An alternative is for an appointment for pre-assessment to be sent to the patient after the out-patient appointment. A date for surgery will be agreed between the patient and the unit at this appointment. It should be made clear in the letter that their surgery is dependent on successful pre-assessment and brief details should be given as to what pre-assessment entails.

Aims of pre-assessment

The aims of pre-assessment can be divided into five sections. The process originally evolved in order to 'screen' for fitness for general anaesthesia, but has now developed to include psychological care, information-giving, discharge planning and health education. Each component is of equal importance, both for the welfare of the patient and for the efficiency of the DSU.

Fitness for general anaesthesia

As mentioned earlier, the anaesthetist is often not able to personally assess all day patients before the day of surgery, and this inevitably means that on admission some patients are found to be unfit for anaesthesia. This causes great inconvenience to the patient, who will have made detailed arrangements to accommodate surgery, for example, arranging time off work, finding a carer and organising transport. The patient may also have undergone considerable anguish over the impending surgery and may now feel 'let down', and the knowledge that he or she is 'not fit for anaesthesia' may cause further anguish. Regrettably, there is often not the time to counsel patients on these aspects.

There are also cost implications for the unit. An operating 'slot' has been wasted and the operating list has one (or more) case less than planned, which, obviously, does not maximise resources.

Occasionally, a patient may be deferred by the anaesthetist because the results of essential pre-operative tests are not available, or the results may be available but have not been checked. Where the findings of, for example, blood tests indicate that medical intervention is required, the day of admission is, clearly, too late for this to be instigated.

Before nurses take on the screening role, a protocol and concise guidelines must be written, stating who should pre-assess and the training required, and the criteria for acceptance for day surgery must be agreed with the senior nurse on the DSU and a consultant anaesthetist. Parameters for acceptance must be agreed, as must the action to be taken if a nurse feels a patient is 'borderline'. Any age limits for patients must be clearly defined and the social criteria agreed. Surgeons should also be involved in the planning of a pre-assessment clinic as they make the initial decision as to suitability of the patient, and some guidance should be laid down as to the types of surgery they are prepared to perform as a day case. It must be agreed by all parties that the nurse has the authority to decide that a patient is not suitable for day surgery despite referral from a surgeon, and is able to initiate treatment which would enable the patient to attend as a day case at a later date. The community nurse liaison service should be involved in the planning and also, if possible, a GP representative. Guidelines must be issued by the consultant anaesthetist as to which patients are deemed suitable for day surgery following the ASA guidelines, and these should be agreed by all the anaesthetists involved in day surgery. Pre-operative investigations need to be agreed and that they should be undertaken by the nurse at the time of pre-assessment. It must be stated in the DSU's policy that no patient will be accepted for surgery unless they have been fully pre-assessed, and all users must agree to this.

Physical and psychological assessment

For the nurse to accurately assess a patient's fitness for anaesthesia, certain physical observations are made. There are two important aspects to the process of carrying out a physical assessment of a patient. The first is the systematic and comprehensive gathering of clinical data. The second is the process and ability to interpret these data.

Using cognitive skills, the nurse notes the posture and demeanour of the patient – is he or she comfortable or in pain? When responding to questions does the patient demonstrate clarity of thought or appear to become confused and muddled?

The general colour and integrity of the skin is noted. The nurse systematically assesses all the systems of the body, recording observations and interpreting the findings thus forming a basis on which to plan for admission and subsequent care. Any drug therapy which the patient may be taking is noted.

The skill of the assessing nurse lies not in the recording of this information but in the ability to interpret it correctly. Interpretation of data is the key to successful pre-assessment. It is not sufficient for the nurse to know the guidelines for acceptability, she or he must also be able to recognise and react to potential problems in the care of the patient.

Some medical and social conditions may cause difficulties for the potential day-stay patient:

(a)   *Obesity* can cause difficulty during anaesthesia, therefore attention must be paid to the patient's weight when selecting for day surgery. Because of the patient's size, a larger volume of induction agent has to be used, which results in a more prolonged recovery, and there can also be problems in maintaining a good airway. A large patient is also more difficult to position safely on the table and, therefore, most units will not accept patients with a body mass index (BMI) greater than 30–35. The BMI is calculated by dividing the unclothed weight (in kg) by height (in m) (Royal College of Surgeons, 1992). Some anaesthetists will accept patients with a higher BMI, and professional judgements and opinions must be considered when setting weight limits.

(b)   *Cardiac problems,* such as cardiovascular disease, can cause difficulties during anaesthesia, therefore, all patients who have a history of any type of heart or circulatory system problems must have an electrocardiogram (ECG) recorded. Many units routinely perform ECGs on all patients over the age of 60. If the nurse does not possess the specialist skills necessary to interpret an ECG, the relevant anaesthetist must see it and make the final decision as to whether or not a patient is suitable for a day-case anaesthetic. However, all day surgery nurses can quickly learn how to record an ECG and many develop the skill needed to interpet them and so will be able to reassure the patient. It is the nurse's role to explain to the patient that the ECG is taken as a precaution because day surgery is planned, and does not necessarily mean that a serious condition is suspected. The patient will be informed after the doctor has made a decision regarding his or her anaesthetic, and will also be told if treatment should be undertaken prior to admission. The nurse acts as patient advocate, not only ensuring that the patient understands what is happening but also arranging referrals and acting in the patient's best interests.

(c)   *Controlled disease.* Many anaesthetists are prepared to anaesthetise those with epilepsy and hypertension, providing these conditions are well controlled, either with or without medication, and many units also now accept patients with diabetes mellitus. The nurse must make a careful note of what treatment, if any, the patient takes and may need to speak to the patient's GP for further advice or to request monitoring over a defined period of time so that the patient will eventually be fit for day surgery. It is important to obtain a urine specimen from all patients, as new cases of diabetes are sometimes discovered during a routine visit to out-patients or during pre-assessment.

(d)   *Gastric symptoms.* If a patient describes any history of gastric problems the type of symptoms should be noted carefully as those who suffer from a degree of gastric reflux, particularly when lying down, pose particular anaesthetic problems. Many anaesthetists prefer not to treat these patients as a day case. Others will treat them as long as the patient is given some kind of H2-receptor blocking agent, such as ranitidine. As many patients will describe indigestion-like symptoms the nurse must take care to distinguish between real acid reflux and occasional gastric upset caused by eating rich food or consuming excessive amounts of alcohol.

(e)   *Neck and jaw mobility.* As the anaesthetist must have total control of the patient's airway during anaesthesia, any potential problems should be identified pre-operatively. The nurse should assess the patient's ability to open his or her mouth and if any kind of surgery to the jaw which has resulted in a small bite has been performed in the past, this should be noted and, in some cases, referred to the consultant anaesthetist. Past neck injuries can also cause difficulties for the doctor if the patient has limited movement in the neck and therefore the nurse should ask the patient about his or her neck and back movement.

(f)   *Previous general anaesthetic.* The patient is asked if he or she has ever had a previous GA and if he or she experienced any problems afterwards. It is important for the nurse to know what previous surgery the patient has had and when, as problems such as post-anaesthesia nausea and vomiting could be attributed to a lengthy, old-fashioned anaesthetic. This must be explained to the nervous patient who has had an unpleasant experience previously and is understandably concerned about repeating the experience. Known allergies to anaesthetics or familial conditions, such as scoline apnoea, must also be noted and the advice of the anaesthetist sought.

(g)   *Social considerations.* The name of the adult who will take responsibility for the patient is recorded and it is stressed that the patient must not return to an empty house. The nurse must also take time to explain that this is a precaution and that serious problems are not expected, but that if the patient is not fit for discharge he or she will be transferred to an overnight bed. The effects of anaesthetic on the ability to drive must be carefully explained and the patient warned that he should not drive for 48 hours post-anaesthesia. If a limb is to be operated on, extra care must be taken before resumption of driving and specific advice given depending on the proposed surgery. The nurse checks that the patient has a telephone in the house and that he or she does not live more than about an hour's journey away from the unit. It is useful to know the patient's occupation and also with whom the patient lives so that appropriate post-operative advice can be given.

The nurse assesses the patient's mobility, which gives a baseline for the nurse to work to post-operatively, particularly after limb surgery. When pre-assessing the more elderly patient the nurse should also enquire after the ability of the spouse to care for the patient post-operatively. In some circumstances intervention from social services and the community nurses will be needed to enable the patient to have day surgery and these services can be arranged at the pre-assessment. A patient who normally cares for his or her spouse will usually prefer to return home after surgery and be with their partner rather than endure the worry that a longer hospital stay would bring. It is therefore in the patient's interests to arrange for after-care to be delivered.

Thus, it can be seen that the nurse requires considerable knowledge of anaesthesia and anatomy and physiology to be able to pre-assess effectively. Without this, pre-assessment should not be attempted until any knowledge gaps have been filled.

Many experienced nurses find that their assessment skills, although knowledge-based, rely heavily on their experience. Decisions not to accept a patient may be based on intuition rather than concrete evidence. These 'gut feelings' must not be ignored (Benner, 1985) as the experienced assessment nurse will rarely be wrong.

Psychological care

Patients who are to undergo day surgery often experience anxiety in the same way as if they were to stay in hospital for a couple of days. Many find the prospect of day surgery daunting, as they know that they will have to take responsibility for their own welfare post-operatively. This knowledge alone can cause considerable anxiety, and pre-assessment goes a long way towards reducing this through the provision of pertinent information and education on post-operative recovery. Mitchell (1994) reports that anxiety experienced prior to surgery is not a minor, short-term emotional disturbance, but is the result of a rational fear of a life-threatening event. He goes on to say that information given in the period immediately prior to surgery may not alleviate this anxiety and that psychological care, in the form of advice on analgesia, support requirements and general information, should be given two–three weeks before surgery.

In a study in Ohio, Kempe and Gelazis (1985) found that anxiety levels in ambulatory surgery patients who were interviewed by a nurse more than a week before admission and who had had their initial nursing assessment performed, were considerably reduced. In the group of patients who were not pre-assessed not only was anxiety higher, but they also complained of more discomfort post-operatively than the other group. In most cases, a well informed patient who has been pre-assessed a few weeks before admission for surgery arrives on the unit feeling relaxed, and the post-operative phase goes smoothly as the patient has had sufficient time not only to assimilate information but also to prepare psychologically for all stages of recovery. It is also easier to induce anaesthesia in relaxed patients.

Psychological care can be viewed as the process by which the nurse assists the patient to cope with his or her emotions. This may involve simply listening to the patient or giving essential information.

Information-giving

A well informed patient is calmer, and good pre-assessment is instrumental in reducing pre-operative anxiety. The patient is not taken by surprise by anything that may happen to him or her and he or she is more likely to comply with important instructions (Mitchell, 1994). Patients vary in their ability to cope with stressful situations (Caldwell, 1991) and to assimilate information according to how much they actually wish to hear. Nurses must use their skill in judging how much information each individual patient requires, and must use appropriate language and terminology according to the patient's ability. It can be a mistake to avoid medical terminology with all patients, as some are quite capable of understanding it and may find the use of lay language patronising and insulting to their intelligence. The nurse must be able to assess quickly the patient's level of mental ability.

There is evidence to suggest that reduced pre-operative anxiety, achieved by appropriate information-giving, can reduce post-operative pain levels (Hayward, 1975). Carr (1989) found that, pre-operatively, many patients underestimate the amount of pain they will suffer and that if pre-operative information is inadequate post-operative pain level and anxiety will be increased (Carr, 1990). If a patient is aware that he or she will experience pain post-operatively, and that that pain will be controlled as far as possible, the actual experience of pain is often not as bad as anticipated.

Obviously, for this vital information to have the desired effect, the way in which it is imparted to the patient is important. Mitchell (1994) believes that information supplied a few hours prior to surgery may well be inadequate. It is generally accepted that a formal, structured process involving both written and verbal communication is the preferred method of imparting information and this is easily achieved in pre-assessment. Studies have shown that some people absorb as little as 20 per cent of the information that is given to them during an out-patient consultation. Firth (1991) concludes that the giving of written information is essential for patient compliance.

Instructions vital for the patient's safety are given, and the patient is asked if he or she agrees to comply. In some units the patient is asked to sign to this effect. This formalises the verbal agreement between the patient and nurse that the patient has received the information and is willing to have surgery as a day case. The patient is given starving instructions according to the time of day surgery is scheduled and to the policy of the unit. The nurse must ensure that the patient understands the importance of these instructions and is clear as to what he or she should do.

Specific pre-operative instructions are then given, such as the use of suppositories for anal surgery or the need to obtain some form of support tights for use after varicose vein surgery. The surgery is explained in as much detail as the patient wants and, if the patient desires, he or she is invited to see the operating theatre suite and the DSU. This is particularly helpful for a patient who is expressing concern at the prospect of walking into the theatre to be anaesthetised or who is worried about the lack of a premedication sedative. The patient is asked if he or she has any questions relating to his or her forthcoming admission and is reassured that he or she may telephone the unit at any time with further questions or concerns.

Discharge planning

Although this subject is discussed in more detail in Chapter 6, it is worthy of mention as a vital component of pre-assessment. As has already been described, successful day surgery is dependent on forward planning for the patient's needs after surgery. The criteria laid down for acceptance for day surgery stipulate that the patient has considered the implications that the surgery will have on normal life and routine, and the after-effects of anaesthesia. Pre-assessment is the ideal opportunity for these issues to be discussed between patient and nurse, and the patient is helped to overcome potential difficulties. Because of the time interval between pre-assessment and admission there is sufficient time for specific arrangements to be made, by either the nurse or the patient. For instance, a patient who normally lives alone has time to arrange to stay with a friend or to have a relative stay with him or her for the first 24 hours after surgery. If he or she had not had the opportunity to discuss the options with a nurse prior to admission the decision may have been made that this patient was not suitable for day surgery, or he or she may not even have been put forward for day surgery in the first instance.

Most patients who are to have day surgery are fearful of post-operative pain. At pre-assessment the nurse is able to discuss post-operative analgesia and to advise on suitable products that may be purchased from a chemist's shop. Hayward (1975) found that for patients to be able to deal with pain effectively they need to have specific information before surgery to minimise post-operative pain. Pre-assessment provides this opportunity.

Planning for discharge in a DSU has necessarily to incorporate advice on how to deal with daily living and social activities as well as how the patient will manage his or her pain. Each component of pre-assessment interacts with the other.

Special post-discharge requirements, for instance, care from a community nurse, can be arranged prior to admission. The patient and carer are able to receive specific instructions to assist them both during the post-discharge phase. This has the effect of reducing anxiety about admission and of enabling the patient to take responsibility for his or her own welfare.

Some units operate a telephone helpline for patients discharged from the DSU. Although this is not usually available to the patient until after surgery, the patient is first made aware of this service at the pre-assessment, which again offers a high degree of reassurance.

By creating a collegiate atmosphere between the professional, patient and carer, the nurse enables the patient to deal more confidently with discharge shortly after undergoing surgery.

Health education

This is now seen as a vital part of modern nursing and patients have come to expect that they will receive advice on health issues from nurses. Pre-assessment offers the ideal opportunity for the nurse to adopt and expand this role.

During the course of the physical assessment, certain health issues will almost certainly manifest. Often, the patient confides in the nurse and asks for advice on issues unrelated to the proposed surgery. The nurse should have sufficient knowledge or have the resources readily available to enable him or her to give satisfactory explanations and answers to all questions.

If the patient smokes, drinks alcohol to excess or is overweight the nurse should take the opportunity to counsel on health. Written leaflets are useful to reinforce the verbal information given and the nurse must use tact and demonstrate empathy and understanding when tackling these often sensitive issues.

Documentation

It is vital that all nurses make and keep accurate records of the care they have given (UKCC, 1992). The pre-assessment interview and subsequent planned care must, therefore, be recorded. In an area of nursing where speed is considered important, if not essential, many DSUs do not use care plans, but instead use either a check-list with tick boxes or ask the patient to fill in a questionnaire. However, the fact that a patient is having day surgery does not preclude him from having planned nursing care in the same way he or she would if staying in hospital for a day or two. It can be argued that because in day surgery the care is delivered in a very short space of time, it must be planned even more meticulously than for a stay in hospital. It has long been accepted practice to use a nursing framework to identify, plan and evaluate care needs to predict and control the clinical setting.

This section discusses the use of care plans in the day surgery setting and looks briefly at a framework for nursing that may be adapted for use in the DSU.

The use of a nursing framework in the day surgical unit

This chapter has already ascertained that pre-assessment has five functions. Incorporated into these components is the initial nursing assessment on which all nursing care is based. Every patient is an individual with unique needs and should collaborate in the planning of his or her own care. Pre-assessment facilitates this by systematically identifying potential and actual problems that the patient may encounter during the day surgery experience.

Orem's (1980) self-care nursing model seems particularly appropriate for day surgery nursing. In her theory, she defined a person as a complex organism with differing needs at different phases in the lifespan. These needs are affected by such issues as age, environment and ability to respond to the health needs of the individual. Orem also made it clear that any nursing intervention must be legitimate in that the relationship between nurse and patient is based on the identified need for nursing.

In the concept of self-care, the emphasis is shifted from doing things for the patient to enabling the patient to do them for him or herself, except where that is totally impossible. Thus, it can be seen that this particular framework, with its emphasis on education and self-directed care, is ideal for day surgery and enables the patient to return safely home a few hours after surgery.

Orem described eight universal self-care requisites common to all individuals, which, if compromised, can threaten health and well-being. These are:

- sufficient intake of air (breathing and oxygenation);
- sufficient intake of water (hydration);
- sufficient intake of food (nutrition);
- elimination processes (renal, urological and bowel functions);
- balance between activity and rest;
- balance between solitude and social interaction;
- prevention of hazards to life, functioning and wellbeing;
- promotion of human functioning and development within desired social groups (the desire to be 'normal').

These requisites may be compromised either through age, poor health or submission to surgery. Self-care is not instinctive, but in response to a need, and Orem argues that although all individuals possess the potential ability to care for themselves, not all will be sufficiently motivated. It is here that the relationship between the patient and nurse, mentioned earlier, commences, in the form of either action by the nurse or delivery of pertinent information and advice.

The stage at which an individual is no longer able to meet self-care requisites is described by Orem as the self-care deficit, requiring intervention from either a health care professional, relative or carer. For example, an anaesthetised patient is unable to maintain sufficient intake of air due to paralysis or obstructed airway and, therefore, has a self-care deficit requiring intervention from an anaesthetist.

Once deficits have been identified at the initial assessment, care outcomes that are realistically achievable are agreed between patient and nurse. Evaluation is undertaken by comparing the initial deficit or problem stated and the goal. Any nursing action required is described using one of five methods:

- acting for the patient (doing);
- teaching the patient;
- guiding the patient (assisting);
- supporting the patient (physically and psychologically);
- creating an environment conducive to development and growth.

Using this framework, a simple to follow and effective care plan can be devised, tailored to the needs of the individual DSU (Figure 2.1). This is used as a tool for planning all care the patient will require through to discharge.

Why not check-lists?

A check-list does not encourage detailed enquiry of the patient. It is often devised for the convenience of the medical staff and does not form the basis for nursing care.

Many day surgery nurses appear reluctant to introduce a nursing framework because they believe this to be time-consuming and irrelevant. DSUs are usually very busy, with a rapid throughput of patients. However, it is for this very reason that the use of a framework is recommended. A patient is less likely to feel as if he or she is a commodity on a conveyor belt if time is taken by the nurse for an in-depth dialogue. The patient is confident that his or her needs and feelings are being taken into consideration and as a result feels empowered to state his or her own views and opinions on the care he or she will receive.

To save some time a core pre-assessment form can be devised, which covers those areas common to all day surgery patients. With skill and experience the nurse will find that a framework-based pre-assessment form takes no longer to complete than a check-list but has the advantage of being truly tailored to the needs of the individual patient.

Patient self-assessment forms

Questionnaires designed for patients to complete either at home, at pre-assessment or on the day of admission are used by many DSUs. These undoubtedly save time, but do not usually allow for discussion with the nurse. There is also the possibility of a patient withholding vital information as he or she does not understand the importance of divulging it.

An effective compromise is to request that the patient completes the form prior to pre-assessment. The nurse is then able to discuss care issues with the patient and plan care appropriately, and any health problems highlighted by the patient may be discussed and the process of information- and education-giving initiated.

Pre-assessment and local anaesthetic patients

Many DSUs with a pre-assessment policy do not pre-assess patients who are to have their surgery under local anaesthetic (LA). These patients have either elected not to have general anaesthetic (GA) or are not fit enough to have GA as a day case. This decision is based on the fact that medical screening for fitness for LA is not required. This policy does, however, have implications for the patient.

	PRE-ASSESSMENT	POST-OPERATIVE ASSESSMENT
1. AIR/PREVENTION OF HAZARDS	Pulse: BP:	Pulse: BP:
History of: Cardiovascular disease Hypertension Chest disease Smoking Epilepsy Hepatitis/Jaundice Drug abuse Neck injury/jaw immobility Previous Anaesthetics Allergies ECG recorded Blood tests taken:	Peak Flow: Yes/No FBC / U&Es / LFTs / TFTs / HepB / Gp&S	Time back on ward: Condition: Pain Score: Analgesic: Wound / PV / PR bleeding:

2. WATER/FOOD/ ELIMINATION
 	
Medication taken:
Indigestion/Reflux
Diabetes
Alcohol
Weight
Height
Diet
Urinalysis
	BM stix: at
	          units / week
	         kg
	        cm BMI:
	Stop fluids at: Food
		Taking water / water by bedside
		Nausea / vomited

3. SOCIAL INTERACTION Name of carer Transport home Type of accommodation Toilet Community nurse Like to be known as Occupation Convalescence required	Car / Taxi upstairs / downstairs / both visit / phone call / twilight	Carer with patient: Escort coming at:
4. MOBILITY Needs help with Aids Back problems	Full / partial / severely limited	On trolley / chair C.W.S.
5. PROMOTION OF NORMALITY		
6. AGREEMENT I understand the need to comply with all instructions I have been given and agree not to drive, operate heavy machinery or sign legal documents for 48 hours after a general anaesthetic.	Signed (patient) .... RGN..................................... Date......................................	RGN... Date...

Figure 2.1: Day surgery care record

NURSING ACTION	EVALUATION	SIGNATURE
Patient to be fit for discharge by................	Assessed fit for discharge by RGN:	
Monitor pain level and give analgesia as required. Check wound / PV / PR loss at................	Pain score: Analgesia given / refused: TTO analgesia explained: Wound / PV / PR bleeding:	
Check blood group...................	Anti-D given: Yes/No	
Mr / Mrs / Ms................................. must / should tolerate diet / fluid by discharge	Has / Has not tolerated diet / fluid	
Mr / Mrs / Ms................................. should pass urine by discharge	Has / has not passed urine	
Give full written and verbal advice to patient and carer	Give full written and verbal advice to patient and carer	
Arrange C/N visit Arrange sick certificate / give advice	C/N arranged and explained to patient. Sick certificate arranged / advice given	
Teach use of crutches / arrange to be seen by physio before mobilisation Patient must be safely mobile by discharge	Patient walking safely with/without crutches Patient up and about walking safely	
	Patient appears relaxed / anxious / distressed	
	Time discharged............................... O.P.A.. G.P.'s letter..................................... TTOs given...................................... R.O.S. arranged for......................... Signed RGN.....................................	

Reproduced with permission of Worthing and Southlands Hospitals N.H.S. Trust.

To the patient, any surgery is traumatic regardless of the type of anaesthetic that will be used. Those who are to have LA will not have had the benefit of receiving reassurance and information from a nurse or other professional pre-operatively. Also, some patients find the very idea of being awake during surgery too frightening to comprehend and without the psychological support that pre-assessment provides may suffer from extreme anxiety prior to admission. This often results in the nurse having to spend extra time with the patient on admission to provide reassurance, impart vital information and attempt to alleviate anxiety.

When patients who are to have LA are not routinely pre-assessed, well written and comprehensive information leaflets need to be devised. These must be sent to the patient at least a week prior to admission so that the patient can read and assimilate the information and telephone the unit if he or she has any queries. The leaflet should cover all aspects of the proposed surgery and state expected outcomes and convalescence required. Many patients believe that because their surgery will be performed under LA it is 'minor', and they may not realise that, surgically speaking, a hernia repair performed under LA is identical to one performed under GA, and that they will require exactly the same amount of after-care.

The ideal solution is to pre-assess every patient who is to have day surgery regardless of the type of anaesthetic to be used. However, in today's climate of restricted budgets and nurse shortages it is clear that this is often not a practical option. Managers should recognise the importance of pre-assessment and secure sufficient finance for the DSU to be able to offer the same high level of care and support to all patients.

Where this is not possible, an acceptable alternative is for a nurse to telephone LA patients prior to admission. The patient is able to discuss worries and anxieties and the nurse is able to plan any post-discharge support that may be required. Patients worry over the apparently trivial issues, such as whether or not they need to bring night-clothes. By telephoning, the nurse is able to allay these fears. This system is time-consuming for the nurse, but the needs of the patient must be of paramount concern. All day surgery patients have the right to be well supported and informed.

Advantages and disadvantages of pre-assessment

The advantages of pre-assessment for both patients and professionals may seem obvious. However, they do need to be weighed against the disadvantages when considering setting up a pre-assessment system for the DSU.

Patient's perspective

Advantages

Undoubtedly, the main advantage for the patient is that he or she arrives for surgery informed and prepared, both physically and psychologically. He or she has received information about the surgery, has had the opportunity to prepare for convalescence and has met some of the staff. It is unlikely that the surgery will be cancelled at the last minute because the patient has been 'screened' for medical fitness. The patient's experience of pain is less than anticipated, as described earlier. The patient has received written information, which is explained by the nurse face to face. Written information should never take the place of the nurse imparting this information face to face, but is a tool to reinforce verbal information and for the patient to refer to once at home. Specific leaflets for each type of surgery performed are also of invaluable help to the patient.

Disadvantages

For those who are committed to the concept of pre-assessment it may seem hard to comprehend that there are any disadvantages for the patient. However, a criticism frequently levelled at pre-assessment is that the DSU is requesting the patient to make another trip to the hospital. For some patients this can pose difficulties if they do not have transport readily available, and some may even struggle to afford to pay extra fares to and from the unit. Many patients are at work and may face problems in having time off on up to three separate occasions (out-patient consultation, pre-assessment, day of surgery).

If the unit adopts a flexible attitude, these potential problems can be largely overcome. One way is to incorporate pre-assessment with the out-patient consultation, but where this is not practical or possible the patient is invited to attend for pre-assessment on another occasion. Patients who receive income support may claim reimbursement for their fares to and from hospital, and help and advice must be readily available for these patients. Appointment slots for early in the morning or late afternoon assist those patients who work and in some exceptional cases where the patient is known to the unit it may be possible to pre-assess over the telephone. The benefits of pre-assessment far outweigh the disadvantages of another journey to the unit and in a study performed at the author's unit, 90 per cent of patients asked, stated that they felt pre-assessment had been very helpful and that they would be happy to attend again.

Professional's perspective

Advantages

From the perspective of the health care professional, pre-assessment is instrumental in ensuring the smooth running of the unit. All patients are fully prepared for surgery, so on the day of the operation there is no need for routine blood tests to be performed and all results are to hand for the medical staff to peruse. There are, therefore, no delays on the day of surgery. All patients will have arranged transport home, resulting in fewer delays in discharge, which can result in 'clogging up' of beds. Patients arrive on the unit with necessary clothing; this has cost implications if it is not necessary to provide, for example, a dressing gown for every patient. They will have known not to wear make-up or jewellery, so time is not wasted removing make-up or locking away valuables. Patients who have attended pre-assessment are less likely to fail to attend on the day of surgery, improving the efficiency of the unit.

Baseline observations of vital signs will have been recorded at pre-assessment and the initial nursing assessment completed, saving even more time for the nurses, which can then be devoted either to those who have not been pre-assessed because they are to have local anaesthesia or to the nervous patient who, despite having attended pre-assessment, is still in need of some psychological support.

As mentioned earlier, pre-assessment plays a large part in the reduction of pre-operative anxiety and this can make the induction of anaesthesia easier and smoother.

Disadvantages

There are some drawbacks to pre-assessment. At least 20 minutes per patient has to be allowed to pre-assess thoroughly. A DSU with two operating theatres and about 10 beds treats around 5,000 patients per year, over half of whom will be having general anaesthesia and require pre-assessment. About 10 per cent of these will fail pre-assessment and have to be replaced by another patient. This means that about 3,500 patients attend for pre-assessment every year, which works out at about 10–15 per day. This considerable workload removes a nurse from the ward team for long periods and must be considered when setting nursing staff budgets.

Some units employ one nurse solely for pre-assessment. This may work well in terms of not having to remove a nurse from the ward team, but pre-assessment can become monotonous and boring for the nurse. Even though all nurses know that communication with patients is absolutely vital, after several days of saying more or less exactly the same things to patient after patient, the nurse begins to forget what has been said to whom and mistakes and omissions can be made. Therefore, a system where several nurses are trained in pre-assessment so that some kind of rota can be devised is preferable. This ensures that no one nurse reaches 'burn-out' and that all patients are pre-assessed by a competent, enthusiastic practitioner.

From the professional's point of view, the psychological and practical benefits of pre-assessment far outweigh the disadvantages.

Training of pre-assessing nurses

It is a mistake to believe that any registered nurse (RN) can pre-assess a day surgery patient effectively. A high level of knowledge of the systems of the body and how to assess a patient effectively is needed. If pre-assessment is to be established, a system of training must be instigated. Where it is well established, adequate training must be given to all new nurses and a system of updating provided for those already pre-assessing.

New day surgery nurses

Many nurses new to day surgery find the prospect of pre-assessment quite daunting and require considerable support while they learn the technique. Indeed, some nurses consider the practice of being able to decide who will or will not attend for day surgery depending on medical fitness beyond their remit as a nurse. However, the United Kingdom Central Council for Nurses, Midwives and Health Visitors (UKCC) in *Scope of Professional Practice* (1992) states that nurses may undertake any task for which they have been properly trained, supervised and assessed as competent, and under the Post-Registration Education and Practice (PREP) requirements from the UKCC all nurses have a responsibility to develop both professionally and educationally and can expect to be given support and guidance from peers. As long as a nurse is not expected to pre-assess a patient without having received structured training and good support from colleagues, all RNs should be able to pre-assess and gain immense satisfaction from performing this role.

Before a nurse begins to learn how to pre-assess she or he should possess sound knowledge of the systems of the body, and have some knowledge of anaesthesia. For this reason newly qualified nurses are not always ideal for day surgery, as some previous experience on either a general surgical or medical ward or in the operating theatre does put the nurse at a considerable advantage. Pre-assessment should be the last day surgery skill that the new nurse learns after rotation through the theatre, recovery and ward areas. To expect a nurse to be able to explain a procedure that she or he has never seen, or to describe the day of admission when she or he has never worked in the ward area is not only unfair to the nurse, but also compromises the care and service the patient receives.

In some DSUs all new nurses spend their first six months divided between the theatre and ward areas. Although they do not become competent in either area in that time, they do have an overview of the type of work done in the unit and will have received a small amount of instruction in anaesthetics, surgical techniques and care of the day surgical patient. A mentor or 'preceptor', who oversees their development and ensures that all objectives are reached and that the nurse receives instruction, will have been nominated.

When training for pre-assessment, the first step is for the process to be fully explained, and the learning nurse must also read the protocol and guidelines for pre-assessment and gain a thorough understanding. A good understanding of the nursing framework that is used must be established and then the nurse can begin to 'sit-in' on pre-assessment clinics (always with the permission of the patient). It is desirable for the nurse to listen to as many different members of the nursing staff as possible, as all nurses will develop their own style of pre-assessment, and as long as all aspects are properly covered there is not really a right or wrong way to pre-assess. The learning nurse should be encouraged to ask questions about the way in which a particular patient has been pre-assessed as this then fosters an atmosphere of inquiry, which is conducive to learning.

When several assessments have been observed and the learning nurse feels ready, the next step is for her or him actually to pre-assess patients under the direct supervision of one of the senior nurses on the unit. The supervisor will allow the nurse to pre-assess uninter-rupted as far as possible, but will ensure that all aspects are covered and is able to assist the learner if something is forgotten or becomes confused. The supervisor should take care not to take over the assess-ment as, if this happens, the learning nurse will not gain the confi-dence to be able to pre-assess alone.

Maintaining and updating pre-assessing nurses

Once the nurse has been passed as competent, the learning process should not cease. It is up to the most senior nurse on the unit to ensure that standards are maintained and that all pre-assessing nurses are kept informed of the latest developments. As confidence in day surgery grows, the criteria for acceptance will change, and all the nurses involved in pre-assessment must be aware of any changes in procedure. Individual anaesthetists may also develop their own criteria, and any changes must be communicated to the nursing staff so the best care and service can be delivered to patients.

Written standards for pre-assessment should be devised. Although these are usually written by the most senior nurse, all nurses should be involved in the process so that they feel some ownership of the standard. Once standards have been agreed by all parties, the process of audit can be implemented to ensure that all patients are receiving the same care and information when they attend for pre-assessment. By reflecting on their own practice, nurses are able to articulate their contribution to the care of the patient and enter into a more collegiate relationship with their medical colleagues. It is for this reason that the pre-assessors should be involved in the audit process, although help is often required from an outside audit nurse actually to collate the vast amounts of information that will be collected. The subject of audit is discussed in greater depth in Chapter 8.

It is imperative that the nurse is familiar with national and local developments in day surgery and keeps up to date by attending seminars and conferences, and reading relevant articles and texts. Every nurse has an obligation under the UKCC *Code of Professional Conduct* to ensure she or he is competent in the task being performed, and to ensure the safety of the patient. Pre-assessment is a valuable process for good preparation of the patient for surgery, and many areas of nursing other than day surgery have adopted it as a means of achieving well prepared and informed patients.

Summary

Pre-assessment is an essential component of day surgery nursing as it facilitates the good preparation of the patient without impairing the efficiency and smooth running of the unit. It is more than a basic nursing assessment and involves specialist skills from a highly trained nurse. As well as utilising the traditional listening and assessment skills of the nurse there is also the opportunity to learn new skills, such as venepuncture and ECG recording, as pre-assessment encompasses the traditional 'clerking' role of junior doctors. With the recent changes to working hours for junior doctors it is reasonable to assume that this new nursing role will continue to develop, thus providing the nurse with an exciting and rewarding challenge. It offers an opportunity for health education and thorough information-giving, as well as 'screening' the patient for medical fitness to receive a general anaesthetic. Time is saved on the day of admission by both nurses and anaesthetists as all essential information and baseline observations have been gathered. It is a role to which nurses are particularly well suited as, traditionally, patients have always felt more comfortable with a nurse than a doctor as they are not perceived by them to have the same social status (Avis, 1992). Nurses also have more contact with patients and often have better developed communication skills than junior doctors in particular. Although in recent years the medical profession has worked hard to rectify this and to become more approachable – and is largely succeeding – there is a shortage of doctors nationally and many feel it makes perfect sense for nurses to take on the role of 'clerking' the patient for surgery and to make the final decision regarding fitness, both for the benefit of patients and to achieve a smooth running and economic day surgery service.

The British Association of Day Surgery and the Royal College of Surgeons both endorse the concept of nurses pre-assessing day surgery patients and many anaesthetists cannot conceive of the idea of there being no pre-assessment. Successful pre-assessment is, however, dependent on the practitioners being well trained, motivated and informed, and working in an environment of co-operation and dialogue between all professionals. Knowledge should be shared between all, and not be exclusive to the more senior members of staff. If these aims are achieved then pre-assessment will reach its goals of well prepared patients, both physically and psychologically, and a day surgery unit that runs smoothly and efficiently for the good of both patients and staff.

References

Allcock N (1996) Teaching the skills of assessment through the use of an experiential workshop. Nurse Education Today 12(4): 287–292.

Association of Anaesthetists of Great Britain and Ireland (1994) Day Case Surgery – The Anaesthetist's Role in Promoting High Quality Care. London: Association of Anaesthetists of Great Britain and Ireland.

Audit Commission (1990) A Short Cut to Better Services: Day Surgery in England and Wales. London: HMSO.

Avis M (1992) Silent partners: patients' views about choice and decision making in a day unit. British Journal of Theatre Nursing 2(7): 8–11.

Benner P (1985) From Novice to Expert. California: Addison Wesley.

Caldwell L (1991) The influence of preference for information on preoperative stress and coping in surgical operations. Applied Nursing Research 4(4): 177–183.

Carr E (1989) Waking up to post-operative pain. Nursing Times 85(P3): 38–39.

Carr E (1990) Post-operative pain: patients' expectations and experiences. Journal of Advanced Nursing 15: 89–100.

Department of Health (1992) Patients' Charter. London: HMSO.

Firth F (1991) Pain after day surgery. Nursing Times 87(40): 72–76.

Hayward J (1975) Information – A Prescription Against Pain. London: Royal College of Nursing.

Irvine C, White J, Ingoldby C (1995) Nurse screening before intermediate day case surgery. Journal of One Day Surgery 4(3): 5–7.

Kempe A, Gelazis R (1985) Patient anxiety levels. AORN Journal 41(2): 390–396.

Markanday L, Platzer H (1994) Brief encounters. Nursing Times 90(7): 38–42.

Mitchell M (1994) Preoperative and postoperative psychological nursing care. Surgical Nurse 7(3): 22–25.

Orem D (1980) Nursing: Concepts of Practice. Maryland: McGraw-Hill.

Reynolds A, Morgan M (1991) Nurses' satisfaction with patient selection and communication in day surgery. Journal of One Day Surgery 1(2): 10–11.

Royal College of Surgeons (1992) Report of the Working Party on Guidelines for Day Case Surgery. London: Royal College of Surgeons.

Thomas S, Wearing A, Bennett M (1991) Clinical Decision Making for Nurses and Health Professionals. London: Saunders/Ballière Tindall.

United Kingdom Central Council for Nursing, Midwifery and Health Visiting (1984) Code of Professional Conduct. London: UKCC.

United Kingdom Central Council for Nursing, Midwifery and Health Visiting (1992) Scope of Professional Practice. London: UKCC.

United Kingdom Central Council for Nursing, Midwifery and Health Visiting (1992) Standards for Record Keeping. London: UKCC.

Further reading

Hartweg D (1991) Dorothea Orem Self-Care Deficit Theory. London: Sage Publications.

Oberle K, Allen M, Lynkowski P (1994) Follow up of same day surgery patients. AORN Journal 59(5): 1016–1025.

Pearson A, Vaughan B (1986) Nursing Models for Practice. London: Heinemann.

Vijay V, King T, Knowles L (1995) Preliminary experience of a day surgery assessment clinic. Journal of One Day Surgery 4(3): 7–8.

Chapter 3
Anaesthetics in day surgery

Gina Behar-Spicer and Rosemary Mitchell

Introduction

This chapter examines the role of the anaesthetic nurse and the care of the patient undergoing anaesthesia in the day-care setting. It is aimed at those nurses who work within a day surgical unit (DSU) who have little or no knowledge of anaesthetics. The chapter is not designed to be used as an anaesthetic reference, but to give nurses some knowledge of the anaesthetic needs of the day surgery patient. It is hoped that it will foster an interest in anaesthetics and encourage nurses into further study. The chapter is divided into specific areas:

1. Nursing care of the anaesthetised patient and the need for day surgery nurses to have anaesthetic knowledge.
2. Uncomplicated day surgery anaesthesia and drugs commonly used in day surgery.
3. Some complications of general anaesthesia.
4. Regional anaesthesia, and the nursing care of the patient undergoing regional anaesthesia.
5. Conclusions and some topics for discussion.

Nursing care of the anaesthetised patient

Anaesthesia is a Greek term that means without feeling, and general anaesthesia can be defined as a drug-induced unconsciousness with a loss of all sensation. Anaesthesia is provided by the use of a combination of two main groups of agents, intravenous drugs and inhalational vapours. Both can be used for induction and maintenance of anaesthesia, although it is more usual to induce anaesthesia intravenously and then maintain it with the use of inhalational vapours. Induction with an intravenous anaesthetic agent produces rapid anaesthesia, usually in the length of time it takes for the drug to circulate from the point of injection through the venous system to the heart, and thence via the arterial system to the brain, commonly termed one 'arm–brain' circulation time. Once anaesthesia has been induced intravenously, it will only be sustained in this way for a matter of minutes. The anaesthetist then uses inhalational vapour to maintain anaesthesia. Other groups of drugs that are used in anaesthesia are opioids and muscle relaxants. These two groups of drugs will be discussed later in the chapter.

Many nurses have either limited knowledge of anaesthetics or no understanding at all, despite this being a significant area of the day surgery environment. This environment is ideally suited for anaesthetic nurses, as they are able to work in any area within the unit, and provide a resource of knowledge for their colleagues, including the pre-assessment and recovery nurses.

The care given to the anaesthetised patient is quite substantial and complex. The anaesthetic nurse provides the physical, psychological and emotional care the patient requires. Admission to hospital causes high levels of stress (Lazarus, 1976), and it is during induction of anaesthesia that the patient may feel particularly vulnerable. This period of the patient's stay in hospital probably causes the most anxiety, and there is a good argument to support the role of the registered nurse as carer during this time.

During anaesthesia the patient is vulnerable to say the least. The anaesthetic nurse is trained to care for the unconscious patient and assist the anaesthetist during induction, maintenance and reversal of anaesthesia. The nurse needs to have knowledge of the drugs administered, their side effects and their subsequent antagonists in the event that these are needed in an emergency situation.

Correct and safe use of tourniquets and diathermy are essential. Tourniquets, if positioned incorrectly or incorrectly inflated, can cause trauma to tissues, leaving bruising and blistering. There are also some medical conditions, such as sickle cell anaemia, where the use of a tourniquet is contraindicated. Diathermy plates should be in close contact with the skin, shaving the area if necessary, to prevent burns. Safe positioning of the patient is vital, making sure to protect nerves, joints, skin and eyes. The ulnar nerves are particularly at risk.

The nurse monitors the patient's vital signs alongside the anaesthetist, and is able to detect changes and assist the anaesthetist in appropriate action should this be necessary. It is the registered nurse's responsibility to assess, plan, implement and evaluate the individual nursing needs of each patient throughout his or her time in theatre. The more knowledge the nurse has about the patient, the better able she or he is to recognise and address the patient's individual care needs.

At pre-assessment the patient may have divulged information relating to health problems that could compromise their subsequent recovery or aggravate existing conditions, such as previous injuries or operations to back, hip, neck and limbs. The anaesthetic nurse, through the very nature of her training, is able to give effective continuity of care once these needs have been identified. In some procedures the patient may need to be positioned slightly differently in order not to further aggravate existing health problems.

Over the past few years this specialist area of care within operating theatres has been delegated to non-nurse anaesthetic assistants. It is quite possible that the use of non-nurse anaesthetic assistants within day surgery units may become a 'thing of the past'. Non-nurse anaesthetic assistants can only be used within the theatre environment, therefore, they are not cost-effective nor are they flexible in times of staff shortage, because they can only be used in the ward areas in a nursing assistant capacity. Now that productivity and cost containment are the main issues in health care it is beneficial to the unit if all members of staff are multiskilled and able to work wherever they are needed.

It is extremely difficult to change ideas and common practice. However, in order to promote the skills of nurses one must justify why nurses should be chosen above more traditionally used operating department assistants/practitioners (ODAs/ODPs). One reason, as already mentioned, is the cost-effectiveness of nurses in the day surgery environment. Another consideration is that anaesthetic nurses are in the unique position of being able to perform the role of patient's advocate, enabling them to look after the patient's welfare and wellbeing. This is a task impossible to perform when the registered nurse is 'scrubbed' assisting the surgeon. While we acknowledge that ODAs/ODPs are highly skilled and valuable members of the theatre staff, the care that the patient requires from the anaesthetic assistant in the day surgery unit is clearly the responsibility of the registered nurse, and one must also concede that registered nurses have spent three years during their training learning to assess their patients' individual care needs competently and are therefore able to assess the patient undergoing a day-case anaesthetic holistically.

Registered nurses who undertake anaesthetic training gain valuable knowledge of the needs of the patient during anaesthesia. The *Patients' Charter* (Department of Health, 1996) clearly states that during a hospital admission a patient can expect a qualified nurse, midwife or health visitor to be responsible for his or her nursing or midwifery care, at all times. The UKCC *Guidelines for Professional Practice* (1996) state in points 11 and 12, 'The nurse has both a legal and a professional duty to care for patients and clients'. Another extremely pertinent reason for undertaking anaesthetic training is that anaesthetic nursing not only provides a stimulating and rewarding field in which to work, but also ensures continuity of care within the day surgical environment. The skills learnt complement those gained throughout a nursing career.

Why all day surgery nurses should have knowledge of anaesthetics

As day surgery expands, an increasing number of nurses will find themselves working in the field of anaesthetics. Day surgery nurses will need to become multiskilled, and the aquisition of knowledge of anaesthetics will enhance other skills already gained during their training and subsequent career. Within the day surgery environment these skills will give nurses the necessary expertise and confidence to pre-assess patients undergoing a general anaesthetic, as well as caring for the patient recovering from an anaesthetic.

It is becoming increasing common in day surgery units in the UK for registered nurses to pre-assess patients prior to an anaesthetic. Lewellyn (1991) states that the nurse at this time should be observing for any signs that could affect a safe anaesthetic and subsequent recovery. To perform this task effectively it is essential to have some anaesthetic knowledge. Bauckman (1991) feels that pre-assessment should only be done by those holding an anaesthetic qualification. However, it is often not practical for all registered nurses working in the day surgical environment to hold an anaesthetic qualification. It is, therefore, reasonable for the nurse to complete a programme of training and be deemed competent by the manager of the unit. This period of training should, in part, be devised by a senior nurse who is trained in anaesthetic patient care and the teaching should be carried out by those with the necessary training, experience, skill and knowledge. We would also recommend spending time with anaesthetists, and all knowledge gained should be regularly updated.

Knowledge of anaesthetic complications is essential when pre-assessing a patient. The pre-assessing nurse must be able to recognise and foresee impending problems that may occur during anaesthesia. It is essential to know how to assess a patient's airway. The nurse should observe whether there is full range of movement in the neck, rigidity or protrusion of the jaw, and understand the implications for the patient if this is so. These problems could interfere with initial induction of anaesthesia, as well as with the maintenance of a safe airway. The assessor must also have knowledge of specific allergies to substances given during an anaesthetic, as well as the relevance of family-related disorders, such as suxamethonium apnoea and malignant hyper-pyrexia (these will be explained in greater detail later in the chapter).

The English National Board's definition of the anaesthetic nurse is: 'Anaesthetic nursing is defined as the care and management of the patient prior to, during and recovering from anaesthesia in any area where anaesthetics is given, either hospital or community'. The recog-nised anaesthetic course is ENB 182, and this has been the training of choice for most theatre departments and DSUs so far. It is a six-month critical care course in anaesthetic nursing. During the six months of training the nurse will work with a trained anaesthetic assistant (nurse or ODA/ODP) learning all necessary practical skills that are required within all specialties in operating theatres. She or he will have to meet certain standards within the clinical area as well as achieving academic requirements. The course provides the nurse with knowl-edge of the underlying physiological changes that occur when an anaesthetic is given to a patient, and how to monitor the patient during this time. The course also prepares the nurse to care for the patient's physical, psychological and emotional needs throughout the peri-operative period. Recently, the course has become modular, leading to a diploma or degree and one would expect the knowledge learnt and the required standard for clinical practice to remain high.

Uncomplicated day-case anaesthesia

Day-case anaesthesia invariably means the admission of a patient, surgical treatment, recovery and discharge within a matter of hours. This obviously necessitates careful planning on all aspects of care. The anaesthetist, therefore, must try to ensure that the induction, maintenance and recovery phases of anaesthesia are smooth, with the overall aim being the discharge of a patient who is alert, orien-tated and free from anxiety, pain and nausea.

In the UK we have tended to be rather traditional and conserva-tive in our approach to day surgery and have, therefore, been slower to adopt this style of treatment. This is in part due to the lack of insurance pressure to limit in-patient treatment as has been the case in the USA. However, as anaesthetic agents have improved we have been able to see the advent of more patients being treated as day cases. There have been several significant advances during the last decade that have enabled this to occur. One is the introduction of the induction agent propofol, minimising the 'hangover' effect and hastening 'street fitness'; another is the introduction of the Laryngeal Mask Airway (LMA), reducing the need for intubation. Other advances include improved inhalational anaesthetic agents and injectable non-steroidal anti-inflammatory drugs.

Patient selection

The initial patient selection is carried out by the surgeon in the out-patients department. It is becoming more common for nurses to pre-assess patients for day surgery; in some units this is carried out following strict guidelines laid down by the anaesthetic department. Once a patient has been selected and pre-assessed it is then up to the anaesthetist to use techniques that will allow the patient to undergo an anaesthetic and recover successfully to 'street fitness' with a minimum of stress and the maximum of sustained comfort.

It is recommended that general anaesthetic procedures for day surgery should last no longer than 90 minutes and the operation should not be associated with excessive blood loss or severe pain. The criteria used for patient selection in the authors' unit is based on the American Society of Anesthesiologists Classification.

Every patient is classified in one of five groups:

- Grade I: a healthy patient without any pre-existing disease;
- Grade I: a patient with a mild systemic disease;
- Grade III: a patient who has a severe systemic disease that is not causing threat to life;
- Grade IV: a patient with severe systemic disease that is a constant threat to life;
- Grade V: a patient who is not expected to live more than 24 hours whether they have an operation or not.

Most day surgery patients fit into categories I or II, but as anaes-thetists and surgeons are becoming more confident in this field of medicine some patients who fit into category III are becomming acceptable. This may depend on whether or not they have been asymptomatic for a period of three months prior to admission (Urquhart & White, 1989).

Premedication in day surgery

The primary aims of premedication are to reduce anxiety in patients and to aid smooth anaesthetic induction. Premedication may have analgesic, hypnotic and anti-emetic qualities; it can also be prescribed to cause the drying up of salivary and bronchial secretions. Opiate premedication is not usually given to patients undergoing day surgery because opiates can cause drowsiness and emesis post-operatively, which may delay recovery and hinder discharge.

As day surgery patients are increasingly walking into theatre, the use of traditional premedication is best avoided. Gibson (1991) states that being able to walk into theatre will reduce anxiety because the patient is allowed to maintain some control of his treatment. However, the use of premedication should not be dismissed completely, as in some cases it is indicated. Induction of anaesthesia in unpremedicated patients often necessitates using higher doses of induction agent than normal. High levels of anxiety increase production of adrenalin and thereby increase the amount of induction agent needed. Some patients who are very anxious need careful handling, and it has been suggested that the more information the patient receives the less the anxiety he or she will experience (Hughes, 1990; Caldwell, 1991). Thus, it is in the preparation for day surgery that pre-assessment is so important, as it is the time when patients can talk about their fears and be given reassurance. However, it remains the case that a few patients will need some premedication in the form of an anxiolytic given on admission, such as diazepam or temazepam.

Other premedication used in day surgery units includes:

• Diclofenac, a non-steroidal anti-inflammatory analgesic, which can be given orally or per rectum (p.r.). It should not be given intramuscularly because of the risk of persistent pain at the injection site. Pre-emptive analgesia is becoming more widespread within some units.

• Metoclopramide, an anti-emetic, which helps to empty the stomach contents.

• Ranitidine or cimetidine, which stops the stomach producing acid and is, therefore, especially useful for those patients who suffer from acid reflux.

• Antihypertensives, if the patient's blood pressure is above the criteria set by the anaesthetic department on admission.

• Atropine, given orally, can be used in children to help dry secretions.

•   EMLA or AMETOP cream, topical for skin anaesthesia, can be prescribed for application to children's hands to allow painless cannulation.

Anaesthesia

It is common practice for patients to be induced with an intravenous induction agent and then for anaesthesia to be maintained with the use of inhalational agents. During this time the patient's airway is secured by the use of an endotracheal tube, LMA or guedal airway and face mask. The most critical times are at induction and at reversal, much like the take-off and landing of an aircraft. The maintenance stage of the anaesthetic should be relatively uneventful. During this time the anaesthetic nurse assists the anaesthetist in assessment of the condition and needs of the patient. The nurse must be able to act accordingly and assist the anaesthetist should an emergency situation arise.

There are many drugs that depress the central nervous system to produce anaesthesia: sedatives, tranquillisers and hypnotic agents. However, with some of these drugs, the doses required to produce surgical anaesthesia are so large that cardiovascular and respiratory depression may occur and recovery can be delayed for hours, even days. Therefore, only a few are suitable for use routinely to produce anaesthesia by intravenous injection.

Drugs commonly used in anaesthesia

Induction agents

Induction agents are mainly given intravenously and are classified in one of two groups: barbiturate or non-barbiturate.

The ideal qualities of day surgery induction agents are:

1.   smooth, rapid anaesthesia;
2.   no side effects: hypotension, cardiovascular depression, respiratory depression, epileptiform fits, nausea or vomiting, pain on injection, no histamine release and minimal risk of anaphylaxis;
3.   rapid awakening;
4.   no hangover effect.

At present there are no induction agents that meet all of the above standards. However, the development of improved agents has had a significant part to play in the development of day surgery. There are four main induction agents commonly used in day surgery.

Propofol – a non-barbiturate

The Pharmaceutical Division of ICI embarked on a research programme to discover an intravenous anaesthetic induction agent with a rapid onset, short duration of action, lack of cumulation on repeated administration, and an absence of excitatory effects on induction and during maintenance and recovery. Propofol was the drug developed through this project in 1980; it became available commercially in 1986. It has taken over as the induction agent of choice for day-case anaesthesia, as quality of recovery is very good. Propofol can also be used for sedation during procedures. It must be remembered that propofol is not licensed for sedation in children. It has also been shown to be painful on injection and some anaesthetists are concerned about the risks of epileptiform fits post-operatively.

Thiopentone

Thiopentone was introduced in 1934 as one of the first intravenous anaesthetic agents. It is a short-acting barbiturate induction agent. However, early recovery is slow when compared with propofol and the slow elimination of the drug from the body may result in persistent drowsiness for 24–36 hours.

Etominate

This was introduced in 1980 and is the induction agent that causes the least depression of the cardiovascular system. It causes minimal release of histamine so is useful for severe asthmatics. Although etominate is short-acting, it is not often used in day surgery as induction tends not to be smooth.

Methohexitone

Methohexitone is another short-acting barbiturate. When very brief anaesthesia is required this induction agent is extremely beneficial and has proven useful in electroconvulsive therapy (ECT). Cardiovascular depression is less pronounced than with thiopentone. However, with the advent of propofol, methohexitone is now not often used within day surgery anaesthesia. It is associated with excitatory phenomena i.e. hypertonus, coughing and movement.

Total intravenous anaesthesia

Total intravenous anaesthesia (TIVA) is the anaesthetising of a patient with a bolus dose of propofol followed by continuous infusion of the drug to maintain anaesthesia. With this method no volatile or gaseous anaesthetic agents are used, but instead, anaesthesia is provided by drugs given through an intravenous cannula regulated by a syringe driver. It takes longer to anaesthetise the patient, but it is smooth, pleasant and there is no pollution of the operating theatre environment by vapours and gases. Moreover, the patient tends to wake slightly quicker with less 'hangover' effect.

Inhalational agents

These agents enter the body through the lungs. They can be used to induce anaesthesia in place of an intravenous induction agent, and to maintain anaesthesia once induction has taken place. A gaseous induction is generally only used in children, when it may be difficult to gain venous access through chubby hands and feet. However, since the advent of topical anaesthetic creams most anaesthetists now prefer an intravenous induction in children.

Inhalational agents may be gases or liquids at room temperature. The volatile agents are liquids that readily evaporate and are delivered by vaporisers located on the anaesthetic machine. The main vapours currently used in this country are halothane, enflurane, isoflurane, desflurane and sevoflurane.

Halothane

This was introduced in 1956 and was the first of the modern volatile agents. It can be described as a volatile hypnotic agent that is fairly insoluble in blood, thereby producing a rapid induction of anaesthesia, and is relatively inexpensive. It does not contain any analgesic properties. Halothane is generally the agent of choice when anaesthetising children, as induction is smooth and is considered to have a pleasant odour. However, it is gradually being replaced for this purpose by sevoflurane.

The effect it has on the body includes depression of the myocardium and the connective tissues of the heart, hypotension and dose-related respiratory depression. Halothane also sensitises the heart to circulating adrenalin, which may lead to arrhythmias.

Roughly 18 per cent of the halothane is metabolised by the liver and the rest is excreted unchanged by the body. One of its main disadvantages is that it can cause changes in hepatic function, especially when given repeatedly over a short period of time. This disorder is known as halothane hepatitis and, although very rare, can be fatal. Halothane also has the undesired effect of relaxing uterine muscles. Another disadvantage is that it can cause 'halothane shakes' post-operatively. The shivering increases oxygen requirements, which can cause hypoxaemia unless oxygen is given.

Enflurane

This was introduced in the 1970s and contains many properties similar to halothane, including being inexpensive, but it has a less pleasant smell.

The effects on the cardiovascular system are also similar to those of halothane, as it tends to cause falls in both blood pressure and pulse, as well as causing respiratory depression. Another side effect is muscle twitching, especially of the jaw and limbs, so it is best avoided when anaesthetising patients who suffer with epilepsy.

The main advantages enflurane has over halothane is that, firstly, only three per cent is metabolised in the liver and it has not been known to cause hepatoxicity, and, secondly, it does not sensitise the heart to adrenalin. Nevertheless, enflurane has now very much given way to isoflurane.

Isoflurane

This was introduced in the 1980s. It has the advantage over both halothane and enflurane that it does not depress the myocardium, but it does, however, produce hypotension through peripheral vasodilation. If increased doses are given it has the effect of decreasing the blood pressure and increasing the depth of anaesthesia.

Isoflurane is kind to the liver as only 0.3 per cent is metabolised, so it is the vapour of choice for patients with liver disease. It causes tachycardia, but arrythmias are uncommon, and it is considered to cause coronary vasodilation. There has been some concern recently over the use of isoflurane in patients with coronary artery disease, as dilation in normal coronary arteries may reduce perfusion in stenosed vessels producing myocardial ischaemia (Aitkenhead & Smith, 1991). Because of its very low solubility it acts and wears off quicker than both halothane and enflurane and has, therefore, become popular for use in day-case anaesthesia.

Unfortunately, isoflurane is expensive and some price-conscious hospital trusts will not use it and recommend that the anaesthetist use alternatives wherever possible.

Sevoflurane and desflurane

These are two new volatile agents which are currently undergoing evaluation. They are both very expensive and so are not yet widely used in the UK.

Desflurane needs a specially modified vaporiser, which may hinder its popularity for general use. However, recovery times are found to be slightly quicker than for patients given isoflurane (Ghouri, Bodner and White, 1991).

Sevoflurane has been used in Japan since 1982 and induction and recovery times are rapid. It has the advantage over halothane of being minimally metabolised and not causing hepatitis. Sevoflurane is expensive, but when used through a closed-circuit or circle can be cost-effective. It has a pleasant smell and may prove popular in gaseous induction in children, taking over from halothane.

Nitrous oxide

Nitrous oxide was first prepared by Priestly in 1772, but was not used in clinical practice until the 1840s. It is colourless, non-irritant, non-inflammable and non-explosive. It has weak anaesthetic properties and it is difficult to induce anaesthesia without using a hypoxic mixture of 80 per cent or more, but it is a powerful analgesic. When used in equal parts with oxygen it produces entonox, which is used during labour and by the ambulance service for analgesia. The main use of nitrous oxide is as a quick-acting analgesic, and it is also an excellent carrying agent of anaesthetic vapours. However, it does contribute to post-operative nausea and vomiting, as well as being a 'greenhouse' gas. Its use is therefore likely to decline over the next few years as medical air becomes more available on anaesthetic machines.

Analgesics

Analgesics are a group of drugs that relieve pain but do not cause unconsciousness. They are an essential part of a well-balanced anaesthetic and may be given as a premedication, on induction, intra-operatively or post-operatively. The ideal analgesic should reduce early perception of pain and produce few and minor side effects. Analgesia is of paramount importance in day surgery and must have the advantage of being effective and long-lasting. The success of day surgery largely depends on analgesia being effective, as this will promote a feeling of wellbeing in the patient and allow for discharge home.

'Opioid' is a term used to describe a range of drugs that are derivatives of opium, as well as synthetic narcotics, such as fentanyl and pethidine. Large doses of opioid given intra-operatively help to reduce many harmful effects of anaesthetic and surgical stress.

It is in the post-operative stage that some anaesthetists do not give adequate analgesia and some seem unwilling to give intramuscular opioids post-operatively. Many anaesthetists still feel that day cases cannot be given intramuscular opioids because the possible side effects of drowsiness and nausea or vomiting may render the patient unfit for discharge. This is illogical, as these patients are unfit for discharge if they have pain. Therefore, a patient in pain must be given analgesia as soon as possible. Providing the pain is controlled and as long as the patient is kept on the unit for a safe period after injection there should be no reason why they cannot then be discharged.

In the authors' unit, pain is still the main reason for patients being admitted for an overnight stay, so it is essential that the anaesthetist and surgeon do everything they can to provide optimal analgesia. In most patients this can be by a combination of local blocks and non-steroidal anti-inflammatory drugs, thus avoiding the undesirable side effects of opioids. The opioids used commonly in day surgery for post-operative pain relief are morphine, papaveretum and pethidine. As most nurses are aware of the action and side effects of these drugs no further explanation is given here.

Other drugs used in the operating theatres of the DSU are fentanyl and alfentanil.

Fentanyl

This is a synthetic opioid that is derived from pethidine but is more potent. A 0.1 mg dose of fentanyl is equivalent to 10 mg of morphine. It is generally given intravenously at induction or intra-operatively, and takes approximately four minutes to reach its peak effect and lasts for approximately 30 minutes. Fentanyl has little effect on the cardiovascular system, apart from a slight slowing of the heart rate, but is a strong respiratory depressant and these effects may be prolonged.

Alfentanil

This is another synthetic opioid with a potency four times that of morphine, but its duration of action is approximately one third that of fentanyl. This makes it ideal for day surgery procedures that last only a short period of time.

Opiate antagonists

These drugs are used to reverse the actions of opioids, e.g. in severe respiratory depression. The most often used is naloxone (Narcan), which is a synthetic antagonist derived from oxymorphone. The dose is 0.1–0.4 mg. It is effective against virtually all opiates, but although it aids recovery of the patient with respiratory depression, it also antagonises the analgesic properties, leaving the patient without analgesia. Naloxone's duration of action is between 45 and 90 minutes and it may need to be given in repeated doses if large amounts of opiates have been used. The most likely use of naloxone in day surgery is when the duration of the procedure has been shorter than anticipated.

Non-steroidal anti-inflammatories

These drugs produce analgesia peripherally by inhibiting the synthesis of prostaglandins stimulated by pain receptors. However, they also inhibit prostaglandin production in the gastric mucosa and lungs, which can result in gastric erosion or ulceration, or severe asthmatic attacks in susceptible patients. These drugs should, therefore, be avoided in asthmatics or patients with a history of peptic ulceration.

Non-steroidal anti-inflammatory drugs are effective in mild to severe pain, and are especially useful in musculoskeletal pain because of their anti-inflammatory properties.

Commonly used anti-inflammatory drugs used in day surgery are given in Table 3.1. Other drugs commonly used in day surgery are given in Table 3.2.

Table 3.1: Commonly used anti-inflammatory drugs

---

1. Diclofenac: Used for acute pain including renal colic, exacerbations of osteo-arthritis, acute gout, acute trauma and fractures, as well as post-operative pain. It may be given orally or per rectum, and the dose should not excede 150 mg in 24 hours. Intramuscular injection is not recommended as it may lead to persistent pain at the injection site.

2. Ketorolac: Used for moderate to severe acute post-operative pain. It may be administered intramuscularly or intravenously. Dose is 10–30 mg, 4–6 hourly. It is not licensed for use in children and should not be used for longer than two days.

3. Ibuprofen: An analgesic particularly useful in rheumatoid pain, other musculoskeletal and soft tissue pain, dysmenorrhoea, dental pain and fever in children.

Table 3.2: Drugs commonly used in day surgery

Drug	Action	Physiological effects
Atropine	Blocks the action of acetylcholine on the parasympathetic nervous system	Causes tachycardia, secretions of the mouth dry up, also those in the gut and tracheobrachial tree. Smooth muscle of the gut relaxes and there is dilation of pupils
Glycopyrollate	Blocks the action of acetylcholine on the parasympathetic nervous system	Same side effects as atropine but for much longer and there is less tachycardia. Can be pre-mixed with neostigmine
Neostigmine	An anti-cholinesterase drug that increases the concentration of acetylcholine at the neuro-muscular junction by preventing its breakdown. Used for reversal of relaxation caused by non-depolarising muscle relaxants	Causes an increase of peristaltic action, bradycardia and increased salivation, therefore should be given with atropine
Prochlorperazine	Action mediated by blockade by dopamine receptors in the chemoreceptor trigger zone	Usually used in the treatment of motion sickness, migraine and Ménière's disease. Not usually given as a premedica-tion but given post-operatively if nausea and vomiting persists. Does not cause sedation and has minor side effects. Dosage usually 12.5 mg 6-hourly. Slight sedative effect
Metoclopramide	Depresses the vomiting centre in the brain. Dopamine receptor antagonist	Stimulates gastric emptying. Increases the tone of the oesaphageal receptor. No sedative but can cause excitability and restlessness
Ondansetron	Acts centrally on the medulla of the brain. Has likely peripheral effect as well	May cause headaches, dizziness, flushing and consti-pation. The most effective of anti-emetics used but is very expensive
Droperidol	A neuroleptic agent. Action similar to that of prochlorperazine	Causes lack of initiative and disinterest in the environment, but patients maintain intellec-tual function. Has anti-emetic qualities – depresses the chemoreceptor trigger zone. More powerful than metoclo-pramide and prochlorperazine but causes sedation and can produce hallucinations

Muscle relaxants

The earliest muscle relaxant was curare, a substance used by South American Indians to poison arrows. In 1850 Claude Bernard, a physiologist, showed how curare worked on the neuromuscular junction. It was not until 1942, however, that Griffith and Johnson described the used of d-tubocurarine in an anaesthetic to provide muscle relaxation in surgical procedures.

As this group of drugs is not commonly used within the day surgery setting, description of their mode of action will be brief. Theoretically, there are three ways to cause a muscle block. The first is a deficiency block, caused when the nerve impulse does not release enough acetylcholine (transmitter chemical) and fails to produce depolarisation of the motor end plate. Some poisons and drugs, such as neomycin, streptomycin, clostridium botulinus toxin (botulism food poisoning) and the venom from the black widow spider, can produce this side effect. If a person has a severe calcium ion deficiency it may also cause this type of block. The other two categories are depolarising and non-depolarising blocks.

There is only one depolarising muscle relaxant currently in use, suxamethonium (Scoline). This drug was first introduced in 1951. Suxamethonium is structurally similar to acetylcholine (the transmitter chemical) and when it reaches the motor end plate it stimulates the receptors, resulting in muscle fasciculation. Acetylcholinesterase (the enzyme responsible for destroying acetylcholine) cannot hydrolise suxamethonium, therefore a muscle block results. Between 75 and 100 mg are usually given to paralyse a male adult; onset of paralysis will take approximately 30 seconds and will last between three and five minutes. This makes it an ideal agent to use for intubating the patient when the anaesthetist needs only a short period of paralysis. As suxamethonium causes muscle fasciculation it can cause post-operative skeletal muscle pains, which, in some cases, can be very severe.

There is also a condition called suxamethonium apnoea, which affects one in 3000 people and is an inherited disorder. An enzyme deficiency results in the drug not being broken down at the neuromuscular junction. The patient will remain paralysed much longer than expected and the condition is detected by the use of a peripheral nerve stimulator. In these circumstances the patient may need to be re-anaesthetised and ventilated until the effect wears off. If the condition is detected at the end of the procedure, the patient, although paralysed, may be awake and this can be an extremely frightening experience so reassurance by the anaesthetic nurse is of the utmost importance.

If a patient is found to have this condition it is extremely important to make the whole family aware of it and to ensure that all are
tested to see whether they are affected. A simple blood test is all that
is required. Many patients are already aware that they have the
condition and this can be picked up at the pre-assessment interview.
It does not usually mean the patient is unsuitable for day surgery, but
obviously the need to avoid suxamethonium is paramount.

The other group of muscle relaxants are non-depolarising
muscle relaxants. These drugs compete with the transmitter
chemical and when they are in greater concentration produce a
neuromuscular block. They do not produce muscle fasciculation.
They can be reversed by the use of the anti-cholinesterase drug
neostigmine, which prevents acetylcholine being broken down by
acetylcholinesterase. Acetylcholine therefore accumulates and
overcomes the block.

Muscle relaxants are not commonly used in day surgery, as the
type of procedures carried out do not generally necessitate intubation. However, there are certain procedures that still require the use
of muscle relaxants, e.g. laparoscopy. Many anaesthetists prefer to
paralyse and intubate these patients because of the risks associated
with this procedure. Aspiration of stomach contents can occur,
because the patient is inverted in the Trendelenberg position. Also
when the laparoscope enters the peritoneum this can produce vagal
stimulation causing profound bradycardia or even asystole requiring
resuscitation. Another procedure where muscle relaxation may be
required is hernia repair. Many surgeons prefer to have the patient
paralysed as it makes the procedure easier to perform.

Commonly used non-depolarising muscle relaxants are:

- Atracurium – Has no significant cardiovascular effects but
  does cause weak histamine release. Can be reversed by the use
  of neostigmine after 25 minutes.
- Vecuronium – A steroid-based muscle relaxant. The most
  cardiovascularly stable of muscle relaxants. Does not cause
  tachycardia, hypotension or histamine release.
- Mivacurium – One of the new non-depolarising muscle relaxants. Broken down by plasma cholinesterase, but without the
  side effect of muscle pain that is associated with suxamethonium. It has an extremely short duration of action and lasts
  between 12 and 15 minutes.

There are other non-depolarising muscle relaxants such as pancuronium, tubocurarine and gallamine, but these are seldom used in day surgery units.

Laryngeal Mask Airway

Another major advance in anaesthesia within the last decade is the invention of the LMA. This advance has been notable for its usefulness in day surgery. Although developed by Archie Brain in 1981, it was not approved for general use until 1988. Prior to 1988 there were two methods of airway control used by anaesthetists. The first was by intubation using an endotracheal tube inserted through the vocal cords. To do this, a muscle relaxant must be administered to allow the tube to be passed through the chords easily. The second method of airway maintenance used was manually holding an oxygen mask on the patient's face with or without a guedel airway. This technique depended on the anaesthetist's skill in holding a mask to secure a tight seal around the nose and mouth and maintaining head extension. Keeping the airway controlled this way is tiring for the anaesthetist and also means that his or her hands are unavailable for other tasks. This method also offers no protection to the airway, so aspiration of stomach contents is a potential hazard.

The LMA has become popular for delivery of anaesthetic gases from the anaesthetic machine to the patient. The advantages include: it does not interfere with the vocal chords and, therefore, cannot traumatise them; the technique of insertion is easy to learn and there is generally no need to use a laryngoscope, thus preventing possible trauma to both teeth and mouth; insertion does not stimulate the sympathetic nervous system so preventing cardiovascular instability; lastly, there is little stimulation of the patient when they are waking up, resulting in a quicker, smoother recovery.

LMAs have, therefore, become commonplace within day surgical theatres and indeed main theatre suites. Many anaesthetists are now happy to ventilate patients through a LMA, and the manufacturers produce them in a range of sizes suitable for use with all patients, from neonates to large male adults. There are also armoured LMAs available for use in ear, nose and throat, and maxillo-facial surgery. The armoured LMA has a thin metal coil within the tube to prevent kinking.

Some complications of anaesthesia

As already mentioned the induction and reversal stages are considered to be the most hazardous periods of anaesthesia. The hazards that may occur are:

1.   Inhalation of stomach contents (aspiration).
2.   Anaphylaxis, which can vary from minor flushing and mottling of the skin to swelling of the pharynx, breathing difficulties and cardiovascular collapse.
3.   Apnoea or breathing difficulties due to:
      (i)   opiates – causing respiratory depression;
      (ii) partial reversal from neuromuscular block;
      (iii) hypocapnia - low levels of carbon dioxide within the blood. Artificial respiration often washes out the patient's CO_2, so reducing respiratory drive;
      (iv) suxamethoneum apnoea;
      (v)   respiratory obstruction – this is often just due to the tongue falling back, but laryngeal or bronchospasm may occur and both of these can be very serious hazards. In severe cases the patient may need to be re-intubated.
4.   Depression of the myocardium, causing bradycardia, arrhythmias and ventricular ectopics.
5.   Profound hypotension, usually due to the induction agent or volatile agent.
6.   Malignant hyperpyrexia (MH). This, like suxamethonium apnoea, is an inherited disorder caused by an autosomal dominant gene, which, when exposed to trigger agents during a general anaesthetic, creates a 'metabolic storm'. This presents as a progressive rise in temperature of between 2 and 6°C per hour. There is also spasm and muscle rigidity and, unless treated quickly and efficiently, the condition is fatal. The drug treatment is dantrolene, which is reconstituted with water, and the dose is initially 1 mg per kg although this can be increased to as much as 10 mg per kg if needed. There should always be a supply of this drug available in the theatre suite. Trigger agents are known to be:-
      • suxamethonium;
      • halothane, isoflurane, enflurane and sevoflurane;
      • phenothiazines (sedatives);
      • tricyclics (anti-depressants);
      • nitrous oxide.

Any patient who is found to have this problem should be referred to St James Hospital, Leeds, where muscle tests will be performed on both them and their immediate family. (For further information contact St James Hospital, Leeds.) It is recommended that anyone found to be positive wears a Medi-alert bracelet.

Regional anaesthesia

Local, regional anaesthesia has been available since its discovery in 1884, using cocaine. It can be defined as the abolition of feeling in a limited area of the body achieved by the injection of an appropriate substance. Patients will often feel touch or pulling, but not the sensation of pain.

Local anaesthesia is often the preferred option for a patient who has moderate to severe systemic disease, as the alternative would be to give the patient a general anaesthetic and plan for an overnight stay in hospital.

Local anaesthesia has many advantages:

1. It is relatively simple for the surgeon/anaesthetist to administer.
2. The patient remains conscious and therefore retains his or her protective reflexes.
3. Quick recovery from the procedure enables quicker discharge to home.
4. It renders the patient pain-free for discharge.
5. It is much cheaper to treat a patient with local anaesthetic than with general anaesthetic.
6. It avoids morbidity and mortality associated with general anaesthetic.
7. It does not cause atmospheric pollution within the operating theatres.

The most notable advantage of local anaesthesia is the analgesic effect. It has therefore become common practice to administer a local anaesthetic to virtually all patients, either directly into the wound or to the nerves serving the wound area. For the patients this results in a period of complete analgesia following the procedure, although the success of the block is heavily dependent on the skill of the surgeon or anaesthetist who administers it. On the whole, the more experienced the surgeon or anaesthetist, the greater the success (an important factor in maintaining consultant leadership within day surgery).

As already mentioned, post-operative pain is the most common cause of overnight admission in the authors' unit. The day surgery patients who are given local anaesthetic blockade appear to benefit from this enormously, and are generally happy and well adjusted to discharge home. By controlling pain, local anaesthesia has a profound effect on wellbeing (Wildsmith and Armitage, 1993).

There are two main local anaesthetics in common use:

1.   Lignocaine (Xylocaine), with or without adrenalin. Adrenalin causes vasoconstriction and so has the advantage of providing a relatively blood-free field for the surgeon to work in. It also prolongs the duration of action of the local anaesthetic. However, because adrenalin causes vasoconstriction this additive is not recommended for use on digits or other extremities, e.g. penis, as the vasoconstriction can cause tissue damage or permanent damage to the nerves.

2.   Bupivicaine (Marcain). Adding adrenalin to bupivicaine does not particularly prolong its duration of action because bupivicaine has no vasodilatory effects. Its duration of action is longer than that of lignocaine (Aitkenhead and Smith, 1991; Carrie and Simpson, 1993) and it is, therefore, the local anaesthetic of choice for post-operative analgesia.

Common regional procedures performed under local anaesthesia

1.   Excision of minor 'lumps and bumps', e.g. sebaceous cysts, moles, lipoma.
2.   Hernia repair, vasectomy, circumcision, local excision of varicose veins.
3.   Carpal tunnel decompression, release of dupuytrens contracture, shortening and straightening of toes, amputation of digits, etc.
4.   Dental extractions.

Common regional blocks used to enhance analgesia with general anaesthetics

1.   Caudal epidural, e.g. for circumcision.
2.   Penile block, e.g. for circumcision.
3.   Inguinal and femoral blocks, e.g. inguinal/femoral hernia repair,
4.   Mesosalpinx block, e.g. laparoscopic sterilisation.
5.   Ulnar nerve, radial nerve, median nerve blocks at the wrist or elbow.
6.   Ankle blocks.

Care of the patient undergoing local anaesthetic

It is imperative that the patient is fully informed about the procedure he or she is about to undergo. A full explanation on admission will help to alleviate any anxiety the patient may be feeling. Many patients having procedures under a local anaesthetic have been deemed unsuitable for general anaesthesia as a day case because of their physical health. Therefore, any patient entering theatre should have their vital signs monitored, including pulse oximetry, blood pressure readings and three-lead electrocardiograph. It is the responsibility of the registered nurse in the theatre to see that this is carried out. It is also a good idea for a registered nurse to sit with the patient for duration of the procedure, not only to monitor their vital signs but also to give them psychological and emotional support and act as their advocate. The patient may be experiencing pain but be too frightened to say, and the nurse can use her skills of observation to detect any discomfort and relay this to the surgeon.

Epidural

The epidural space is a false space in the spinal column between the dura mater and the ligamentum flavum, which is largely filled with fat and blood vessels. Epidural anaesthesia can be used for day case surgery but is more usually used for chronic pain conditions (mainly sciatic pain). In this situation, the anaesthetist injects a mixture of steroid and local anaesthetic into the epidural space to reduce inflammation of the nerve roots. The local anaesthetic should give almost immediate relief from the symptoms and the steroid should start to work within three to five days, giving relief for up to six weeks. However, it is worth mentioning that at present no steroid preparations are licensed for use in the epidural space.

There has been much controversy in recent years over the complication of this procedure, namely arachnoiditis, which can occur when the steroid preparation (Depo-Medrone) comes into contact with the arachnoid mater. Although this complication is potentially extremely serious and can cause paralysis, it is extremely rare if the epidural is carried out correctly. However, patients need to be aware of this complication prior to signing a consent form.

Other complications of an epidural are:

1. Hypotension due to sympathetic nerve blockade reducing venous return to the heart and causing vasodilatation.

2. Retention of urine due to lack of bladder sensation. This is generally the result of large dosages of local anaesthetics being used in the lumber region.
3. Pruritus can occur if opioids are injected into the epidural space.
4. A severe headache can develop if the dura mater is punctured and the patient loses cerebrospinal fluid.
5. The patient can suffer backache for up to 48 hours.
6. An epidural abcess or haematoma can result due to bad aseptic and faulty technique, although this is extremely rare.
7. Respiratory muscle paralysis can occur if the block ascends too far. Intercostal paralysis will render the patient unable to cough.

Nursing care of the patient undergoing epidural analgesia

It is imperative for the nurse to have explained the procedure to the patient so that he or she is aware of what to expect during and post-epidural. As in all procedures carried out while the patient is awake and aware, there may be anxiety and fear. The anaesthetic nurse can help to alleviate these fears, and thus allow the procedure to be performed quickly and effectively without undue trauma to the patient.

Before the procedure the patient's vital signs must be monitored and recorded. A cannula is inserted in the back of the hand to allow intravenous access, should the need arise. Ephedrine and/or intravenous fluids may need to be given in cases of hypotension. The patient's vital signs should also be monitored during the procedure. The anaesthetic nurse should watch for any changes in the blood pressure, three-lead electrocardiograph and pulse oximetry recordings and report them to the anaesthetist immediately. A second nurse should sit with the patient to give support and encouragement, and should use his or her skills of observation to detect any changes in the patient, such as signs of stress, anxiety, pain and discomfort.

After the procedure the patient is positioned on his or her back with just one pillow beneath the head. Before the patient is taken to the recovery room a blood pressure reading is taken to ensure there has not been a dramatic drop. In the recovery room the patient's vital signs must be monitored. On return to the ward the patient is encouraged to remain lying down for approximately one hour and then gradually sit up in stages, which usually takes a further hour. If the patient remains symptom-free, he or she is allowed to get up, get dressed and sit in a chair. On discharge, full information of post-operative care should be given, as well as signs and symptoms to be aware of, and who to contact if the need arises.

Conclusion

It has not been possible to cover every aspect of anaesthetics in this chapter, as it is such a huge area of medicine. However, it is hoped the reader will have gained an overview of this specialty.

Day-case anaesthesia carries with it the same complications as in-patient anaesthesia, therefore all the resuscitation equipment within a DSU must be the same as that in main theatre suites. Other emergency equipment, such as 'difficult intubation' equipment, must also be on hand because the majority of patients suitable for day-case anaesthesia will be young and healthy and this may, therefore, be their first general anaesthetic experience.

One point of discussion is the question of whether to anaesthetise in theatre or in the anaesthetic room. Anaesthetic rooms in many day surgery units have, in recent years, become used solely as storage rooms for anaesthetic and emergency equipment. Most are not equipped with appropriate monitoring equipment, and cost constraints have prevented the purchase of the additional equipment needed to monitor patients during the induction phase of anaesthesia. Therefore, it has become common practice to anaesthetise patients in the theatre itself, where all necessary monitoring equipment is available. Another good reason for anaesthetising in the operating theatre is the need to keep the period of general anaesthesia as short as possible for the patient. This also optimises the throughput of patients. The one possible exception to anaesthetising in the operating theatre is with children, because for them the anaesthetic room can be a much less frightening environment than the theatre.

Now that patients are being encouraged to walk into the operating theatre, nurses must not lose sight of the high levels of anxiety this may cause. Attaching the monitoring equipment is another source of anxiety. Therrien (1990) reminds us that it is important to inform the patient exactly what the monitors are and what function they perform.

Some units do use anaesthetic rooms for induction of anaesthesia. Where this is the case the anaesthetic rooms should be pleasantly decorated and patient friendly, especially if children are to be anaesthetised in them, as this can help to relieve anxiety. However, Porteous and Tyndall (1994) found that in their experience the majority of patients prefer to walk into the operating room rather than be wheeled on a trolley into an anaesthetic room.

The development of improved anaesthetic agents has undoubtedly had an important part to play in the development of day surgery. The quest for the 'perfect' anaesthetic induction agent continues and the patient's psychomotor responses comparing the various agents currently available will continue to be measured. However, no matter how rapid the initial recovery, it remains usual for patients to be discharged home approximately three hours post-operatively. After this period of time, it is debatable whether patients anaesthetised with different vapours or indeed TIVA show any marked difference in level of consciousness from the nurses caring for them or the relatives taking responsibility for them at home.

Day surgery anaesthetics need to be smooth, uneventful and with rapid recovery to 'street fitness'. The unnecessary use of opioid premedication and the use of anaesthetic induction and mainte-nance agents which aim to minimise 'hangover' effects have been discussed. The patient must be given sufficient analgesia and be able to understand and comply with all pre-operative and post-operative instructions. Morbidity such as nausea, vomiting and dizziness must be minimised.

When a patient has been discharged from hospital after being given powerful anaesthetic drugs, the patient must be aware of how they will feel. Any impairment of his or her ability to function normally may not be easily noticeable. It is the responsibility of the registered nurse to inform the patient and his or her carer how the patient is likely to feel, and that he or she must not be left alone for at least 24 hours post-operatively. The carer must also be given explicit instructions on how to care for the patient and where to get help if needed.

Nursing within the field of anaesthetics carries enormous respon-sibilities towards the patient. Skill and expertise are required not only in the clinical aspect of the tasks involved, the nurse must also be empathetic to the emotional needs of the patient. Anaesthetic nursing is a stimulating field of specialism and it is hoped that more nurses will express an interest in this field as many operating depart-ments have lacked the presence of anaesthetic nurses in recent years. Day surgery units are ideal areas for anaesthetic nurses, whose knowledge is invaluable in pre-assessment clinics. They can deal with many of the queries relating to anaesthetic problems found at pre-assessment, therefore reducing the need to call the anaesthetist for minor queries.

It remains the fundamental aim of modern day surgery that the care delivered to the patient should be of the highest quality. Unfor-tunately, the care given to patients on general wards who are sent home the same day is often not of the same standard. With further advances in anaesthetic techniques and further cost constraints it seems sensible to assume that day surgery will continue to increase. At the same time, nurses working within day surgery units and those with specialist skills in anaesthetics must continue to strive for high standards of patient care.

References

Aitkenhead AR, Smith G (1991) A Textbook of Anaesthesia, 2nd edn. London: Churchill Livingstone.

Baukman D (1991) The ODA as a patient's advocate. Technic 95.

Birrell J (1988) Managing anxiety. Professional Nurse 3(7): 243–246.

Caldwell LM (1991) The influence of preference for information on pre-operative stress and coping in surgical operations. Applied Nursing Research 4(4): 177–183.

Carrie LES, Simpson PJ (1993) Understanding Anaesthesia, 2nd edn. Oxford: Butterworth-Heinemann.

Department of Health (1992), (1996) The Patients' Charter. London: HMSO.

Gibson C (1991) A concept analysis of empowerment. Journal of Advanced Nursing 16(3): 354–361.

Ghouri AF, Bodner MD, White PF (1991) Profile after desflurane–nitrous oxide versus isoflurane–nitrous oxide in outpatients. Anaesthesiology 91(74): 419–424.

Hughes J (1990) Stress: scourge or stimulant? Nursing Standard 5(4): 30–33.

Lazarus A (1976) Multi model behaviour therapy. Cited in Bailey R, Clarke M (1989) Stress and Coping in Nursing, 2nd edn. London: Chapman Hall.

Lewellyn J (1991) Short stay surgery: present practices, future trends. AORN Journal 53(5): 1179–1191.

Porteous A, Tyndall J (1994) Yes I want to walk to the operating theatre. Canadian Operating Room Journal 12(2): 15–23.

Therrien S (1990) Patient education. Gastroenterology Nursing 13(1): 54–56.

UKCC (1996) Guidelines for Professional Practice. London: UKCC.

Urquhart M, White PF (1989) Out patient anaesthesia. In Nimmo WS, Smith G (Eds) Anaesthesia. Oxford: Blackwell Scientific Publications.

Whitwam JG (1994) Day Case Anaesthesia and Sedation. Oxford: Blackwell Scientific Publications.

Wildsmith JAW (1987) Three Edinburgh men. Regional Anaesthesia 9: 161–164.

Wildsmith JAW, Armitage EN (1993) Principles and Practice of Regional Anaesthesia 2nd edn. Edinburgh: Churchill Livingstone.

Further reading

Brimacombe J (1993) The Laryngeal Mask Airway. Tool for airway management. Journal of Post-Anaesthesia Nursing 8(2): 88–95.

Davis JE, Sugioka K (1987) Selecting the patient for major ambulatory surgery: surgical and anesthesiology evaluations. Surgical Clinics of North America 67(8): 721–732.

Evans CLS (1991) A Conceptual Framework for Nursing. Newbury PK, CA: Sage.

Green A (1991) Making sense of Laryngeal Masks. Nursing Times 87(10): 36–37.

Hollander D (1994) Gastrointestinal complications of non-steroidal anti-inflamma-
  tory drugs: prophylactic and therapeutic strategies. American Journal of
  Nursing 96: 274–280.
Klepper ID, Sanders LD, Rosen M (1991) Ambulatory Anaesthesia and Sedation
  Impairment and Recovery, 1st edn. Oxford: Blackwell Scientific Publications.
Long BC, Phipps WJ (1985) Essentials of Medical/Surgical Nursing. St Louis,
  Missouri: Mosby.
Wall PD, Melzack R (1989) Textbook of Pain, 2nd edn. London, Edinburgh,
  Melbourne: Churchill Livingstone.

Chapter 4
Theatre nursing in day surgery

Sarah Williams and Jacqui Rollason

Introduction

This chapter describes the surgical techniques most often performed in the day surgery setting. It outlines the role of the theatre nurse, describes the care of the patient undergoing surgery and discusses the special needs of the day surgery patient in theatre.

Only those operations covered in the *Guidelines for Day Case Surgery* (Royal College of Surgeons, 1992) are included here, although many different procedures will be carried out in day surgical units (DSUs), depending on the surgeon's interests, equipment available and the training staff have undertaken.

The range of procedures carried out has expanded as surgeons have recognised that more work can be undertaken on a day-case basis, and as the government, recognising the potential savings to be made and the lowering of the waiting list time, injected a substantial increase of funding into this area. There has been a 30 per cent increase in day surgery cases in the last six years (NHS Management Executive, 1993).

Because of the need for all techniques to be consultant or senior registrar led, it follows that those surgical procedures undertaken must be supported by a consultant who, ideally, is enthusiastic about the concept of day surgery. As units expand it may be possible for visiting consultants to carry out procedures in their own specialties, but this must be well thought through as any problems that lead to in-patient admissions could put the patient at risk. For example, the authors' unit has no ear, nose and throat (ENT) in-patient facility, yet day-case surgery is undertaken in this area, and any complications require the patient's admission to an alternative centre.

In day-case surgery nursing awareness of patients' fears and anxieties is of vital importance and staff must be able to lessen these fears in any way achievable. This may involve simply holding a hand or it could mean giving a full explanation of procedures and answering questions over and over again until the patient is satisfied. If the member of theatre staff who is collecting the patient can introduce herself or himself to all patients before the list commences there will be an instant point of contact and recognition. This is also a good time to ask if the patient has any worries or questions and, if so, to answer them fully. The contact is then remade if the patient is taken through to the theatre by the same member of staff. The patient should have this same nurse close by until they are fully anaesthetised.

Day-case patients have specific needs from a surgical aspect. Surgeons must be skilful and competent to perform the procedure quickly and efficiently, and minimise any post-operative complications. They must also have expertise in such areas as haemostatis, appropriate use of drains, when applicable,and correct use of sutures and dressings. There must be analgesic agents available to minimise pain and discomfort post-operatively, thus producing a fast, efficient and comfortable outcome, with minimal risk of complications. The days of 'watch one, do one, teach one' are over in the medical profession, as can be seen by the accreditation centres now being set up for the newer techniques of laparoscopic surgery. Laparoscopic surgery is a fast growing area and will be discussed later.

The role of the theatre nurse in day surgery

The theatre nurse was the first specialist nurse (Nightingale, 1986) requiring a 'level hand, keen eyes, ever watchful for all that may be required, a mind not easily irritated or confused, combined with the facility of keeping out of the way and still being of the greatest help.' (Francis, 1889, cited in Wicker, 1987).

Historically, nurses cared for patients both pre- and post-operatively in addition to assisting the surgeon during the procedure. But as the number of operations performed increased, so did the number of surgeons; it thus became necessary for nurses to restrict themselves to the intra-operative care of the patient. This trend led to the separation of the operating room nurse from the ward nurse.

Today's theatre nurse is a highly trained, skilled person whose role is complex and difficult to define. Carrington (1991) describes the role as combining the technical knowledge and expertise associated with sophisticated instruments, techniques and drugs in current use, and the basic nursing skills acquired through training and experience that are vital to the care of the patient. Highly specialised knowledge is required in the care and maintenance of instruments and procedures to preserve a safe environment for the patient. The patient is at his most vulnerable in the operating theatre when he is not in control of his own environment and cannot warn, tell or object.

There has been considerable debate (McGee, 1992) about the nature of theatre work and whether the activities that theatre nurses perform can be called nursing. It has been suggested that theatre nurses have almost disappeared behind operating theatre barriers, becoming so engulfed in machinery and gadgetry that they have lost track of the patient and it is often said that a nurse works in theatre to escape patient contact. However, it is precisely because of the nurse's ability to care for patients that there is a place for her or him in theatre.

The day surgery nurse is not only a theatre and anaesthetic specialist but also a practitioner with added day surgery expertise. She or he has all the knowledge and skills of the theatre environment, the added skills needed for recovery nursing, pre-assessment, pre- and post-operative care, and information-giving, and has a total overall picture of the sequence of patient events from the first appearance in the unit until the patient episode is completed. This can be seen as a return to the total care scenario that occurred before specialisation took place.

There are two approaches which can be further taken into account in this equation. Penn (1993) takes the view that nurses should be educated to be skilled in all areas of day-case surgery and be utilised in all areas. Sutherland (1994) argues that unless constantly used, specialised skills are diluted. He believes it is unreasonable to expect nurses to be competent in such differing areas as pre-assessment, pre-operative care, admission, information-giving, recovery, anaesthetics, theatre and post-operative care, in addition to computer skills and management skills, all of which may be required; the 'super nurse'.

The authors believe that the day surgery practitioner should be competent in her or his own area and have knowledge in all other areas, but this will depend on how individual units are managed. Many units rotate staff, whereas others keep specialists in their own areas. Among the most important areas of competency for the theatre practitioner is the pre-operative assessment and, where possible, an informal discussion with the patient on admission. These help to reduce anxiety and enable the patient to be familiar with the nurse from theatre (Hayward, 1975).

The National Association of Theatre Nurses (NATN) states that day surgical nursing care in the operating theatre should be of the same high standard as in-patient care. The nurses' role in the operating theatre is to provide nursing care and safety for the patient. The staff in the operating theatre are a closely involved team whose common aim is the provision of the best possible care for the patient. Each member of the team has a clearly defined responsibility, but each must depend on the others for support and assistance.

The usual staffing for a theatre is three trained staff; in the authors' unit these will be trained nurses, one of whom is anaesthetic trained, one who is allocated to scrubbing and one for circulating. In addition, it is usual to have one health care assistant or operating department orderly.

The scrub nurse

The scrub nurse takes ultimate responsibility for the care of the patient. At the commencement of each session she or he must check the theatre list of proposed operations and ensure that all equipment is available and in working order. The nurse must also check with the ward nurse that the patients have arrived and are fit for operation, and discuss the organisation of the list with the team, e.g. who will scrub up and assist the surgeon, who will collect the patients from the ward, and who will hand over to recovery staff.

The scrub nurse is the member of the team who prepares the sterile instruments trolley and keeps account of the swabs, instruments and needles used during the operation. The scrub nurse needs to be able to anticipate the surgeon's needs, react quickly and have a knowledge of anatomy and operative procedures.

Scrubbing, gowning and gloving must be undertaken with reference to the NATN guidelines and local policies, the aim being to ensure minimal microorganisms on the hands and arms, and correct donning of sterile gown and gloves to maintain full sterility.

Swabs, needles and instruments

One of the scrub nurse's most important jobs is to account for swabs, instruments and needles at all times during an operation, to prevent any foreign bodies being left in the patient, as this could cause subsequent injury to the patient.

Instruments

In most units the instruments will be pre-packed in a central sterilising department. All sets will contain a list of instruments that should be present in that set. Before each case the scrub nurse and circulating nurse must check that all instruments are correct. The scrub nurse must also check that the instruments are in working order, that screws and any loose parts are present, and that diathermy leads and forceps are insulated and intact. Any faults or discrepancies must be noted.

Swabs

All swabs used in theatre contain a radio-opaque marker and are packed and tied in bundles of five.

Counts

All swabs, needles and instruments must be diligently checked by two people, one of whom must be a registered nurse, before the operation begins. The number of swabs, needles, blades and hypodermics is then recorded on the count board and in nursing documentation.

The scrub nurse must remain aware of where all swabs, needles and instruments are throughout the operation. Counts should be carried out at the closure of each layer and before the closure of the skin, and the surgeon must be informed that all is correct.

No swab, needle or instrument should be removed from the theatre until the end of the operation. In the event that a swab, needle or instrument is found to be missing, the surgeon must be informed and a thorough search made. If the lost item is not located an X-ray should be performed on the patient and the incident recorded in the nursing notes and theatre register.

Analgesia

The analgesic cover given intra-operatively is of major importance in day surgery. In the authors' unit, all patients are required to give consent for rectal analgesia, and the drug of choice is the anti-inflammatory drug diclofenac.

Local anaesthesia is infiltrated to the wounds of all general anaesthetic patients. The drug of choice in the authors' unit is bupivicaine, either with or without adrenalin. The scrub nurse must have this available for all cases and ensure it is used by the surgeon.

Regional blocks may also be administered by the anaesthetist or surgeon, e.g. penile blocks, caudal blocks or brachial nerve blocks. This is discussed in Chapter 3.

Skin prep and draping

The skin is always cleaned with an antimicrobial solution. Spirit-based solutions are used on the skin surfaces and aqueous solutions are used on mucous membranes. Pre-operative shaving has been shown in several studies to contribute to post-operative wound infection (Freshwater, 1992). Despite the research, most surgeons continue to insist on pre-operative shaving. Alternative methods, e.g. depilatory creams, can cause adverse skin reactions. AORN (1987) recommended shaving as near to time of surgery as possible, i.e. in theatre.

The site of incision and the surrounding area are cleaned. The method of cleaning is to start at the incision site and clean outwards, never going back towards the incision site with the same cleaning sponge. Cleaning should always end at the dirtiest area, e.g. the umbilical or groin area.

Sterile drapes are used to create a sterile area around the operative site. When cotton or linen drapes are used a moisture-proof layer must be placed underneath the drapes. Disposable drapes are usually reinforced with a moisture-proof substance so they repel blood and water. Disposable drapes are now being more widely used, particularly for orthopaedic cases where any infection introduced to bone is extremely serious. These drapes are designed and folded for easy use. The sterile drape must be kept higher than waist level until it is positioned. The nurse's gloves must be well protected by folding the corners of the drape around the hands so that the drape can be placed without contaminating the hands.

If a drape is positioned wrongly it cannot be repositioned, it must be discarded and replaced. Towel clips are used to hold the drapes in place; care must be taken not to nip the patients skin with the towel clips. Once the towel clips are positioned they must not be repositioned. Alternatively, steridrapes (a clear adhesive plastic drape) can be used to exclude the need for towel clips and provide further sterility.

Draping for specialised operations, such as those in lithotomy position, will include leg drapes and perineal sheets. For ENT and dental surgery head towels must be available.

During and after the operation

Once the patient is fully draped, diathermy and suction, if used, must be securely positioned within easy reach of the surgeon. All instruments must be handed in such a manner as to be instantly usable by the surgeon. All instruments with a ratchet must be handed closed. Special care must be taken to pass scalpels in the appropriate manner so that neither the nurse or surgeon are in any danger of accidental injury. Scalpels must be placed in a kidney dish when not in use. When passing scissors the surgeon must know that they are scissors, this is especially important when anticipating need, not having been asked. Diathermy forceps and points must be regularly cleaned to be effective.

After the operation the wound area must be cleaned in the appropriate manner, i.e. from the wound out, the dressing of choice applied, inspection for any further blood made and any necessary cleaning carried out.

All drains are sewn in by the surgeon. Corrugated or red rubber drains should have an additional guard of a safety pin and further strapping to make it secure. It is especially important to ensure suction drains are properly secured and vacuumed.

If the patient is to be returned to the ward on the same trolley that was used as the theatre table, the sheets and blankets must be clean and dry. This may mean changing the sheet in theatre.

Dressings

The theatre team must be aware of the different types of dressings available and the surgeon's preference. The dressings most commonly used are small elastoplasts for tiny incisions, adhesive dressing with a non-adhesive absorbable centre, e.g. Mepore or Primapore, and clear adhesive dressings where the wound can be observed, e.g. Tegaderm or Opsite.

Pressure dressings are used for areas at risk from capillary bleeding and subsequent bruising, e.g. the breast. A wound dressing is applied, followed by gauze, padding or both, and this is secured by several long lengths of stretched adhesive bandage.

Whenever bandages are required, their correct application is important. When applied to limbs, a layer of padding material, e.g. Orthoban, is applied before a crepe bandage. The tension of the bandage must be sufficient to apply pressure but not to constrict blood vessels. Fingers and toes must always be exposed and colour and mobility noted.

Plaster of Paris must be available, with warm water to moisten the plaster. It is used for maintaining the position of a limb post-operatively in orthopaedic cases and must allow full movement of the joints above and below the cast.

Sutures

The range of suturing materials is vast and growing. For day surgery the use of absorbable sutures is on the increase. This negates the need for removal. Subcuticular suturing with an absorbable suture is recommended by the Royal College of Surgeons (1992) in *Guidelines for Day Surgery*.

Absorbable sutures are broken down by enzymes or by hydrolysis. The range available includes plain and chromic catgut, dexon, vicryl, monocryl and p.d.s. Chromic catgut is plain catgut that has been immersed in chromic salts to delay absorption. Dexon, vicryl and p.d.s. are manmade absorbable materials. The length of absorption, surgeon's choice and site of operation will determine the material used.

Non-absorbable sutures, which remain permanently or until removed, include nylon, and nylon derivatives, prolene, Novafil, gortex and silk.

Sutures that are stored in solution, e.g. catgut, should not be allowed to dry out as this causes loss of strength. Some sutures require straightening, e.g. prolene and catgut. This is done by careful pulling, without putting undue strain on the needle suture connection. A clip should be put on the end of nylon materials when used to suture the skin subcuticularly to prevent it being pulled through the skin. Catgut may be lubricated when used for skin, e.g. in circumcision.

Ties are used for ligating vessels. These are normally absorbable and of catgut or vicryl. They should be cut into appropriate lengths and presented stretched between the scrub nurse's hands for easy surgical use.

Needles

Needles come in various shapes and sizes, and the type used will depend on the nature of tissue to be sutured. Most needles are atraumatic, meaning the suture material is welded into the shaft of the needle.

In general, round-bodied needles are used for more friable tissues, trocar point where an initial strength is needed, and cutting for skin. Reverse cutting and prime needles are also coming into use. Needles can be straight or have a variety of curves.

Documentation

Documentation is used to provide a record of the care given in theatre. The information must be documented in both the theatre register and the nursing care plan. Both these documents are legal evidence of the care given, and are signed by both the scrub nurse and the circulating nurse, stating that the information is correct.

The register states the patient's name, age and hospital number. The operation performed is entered by the scrub nurse at the end of the case and the register signed. The surgeon's name, anaesthetist's name, type of anaesthetic given and the number of the instrument tray are also recorded.

Additional information that should be added are the specimens sent and tourniquet time. This register is signed by the scrub nurse stating that swabs, needles and instruments were correct at the end of each case.

The nursing care plan provides a record of safety of care given and includes positioning of the patient and positioning of the diathermy plate. It also contains information that is useful for immediate post-operative care, such as skin suture used, dressing used, local anaesthetic (LA) infiltration and any packs or drains in position. Any incidents that occur during the operation, e.g. knocking out of teeth by the anaesthetist or pinching of skin from towel clips, must also be recorded in the nursing notes.

The circulating nurse

The circulating nurse has a duty to the patient, the scrub nurse and the overall smooth running of the theatre. Both nurses will ensure that the theatre equipment is not only present but working efficiently. Diathermy and suction apparatus must be turned on and the safety of all equipment checked. All waste, laundry bags, gloves and gowns needed must be present and a supply of all disposables ready to hand, e.g. swabs, sutures and dressings. If the list to be undertaken is a specialist list all extra requirements must be available, e.g. tourniquets and light sources, and these must be in full working order. Once the theatre is prepared the scrub nurse will scrub while the circulating nurse opens the tray of instruments. All lotions, swabs and extra instrumentation should be near to hand and the circulating nurse must be ready to open these once the scrub nurse has gowned and gloved. Any articles that may be needed, rather than definitely needed, should be either under the trolley or readily available. A count of instruments, swabs and needles is carried out and documented on the theatre board and nursing notes.

At all times both nurses must maintain full sterility, the circulating nurse offering items to the scrub nurse in a manner easily acceptable – not over the trolley. The scrub nurse will take them with an instrument rather than by hand.

In the authors' unit a nurse collects the patients and stays with them until they are fully anaesthetised. Once the patient is anaesthetised the nurse must show the consent form to the scrub nurse and any allergies must be noted. The circulating nurse will check that the scrub nurse is satisfied with all aspects of patient safety, positioning, correct use of arm boards, application of diathermy plates and tourniquet. She or he will keep a close watch on proceedings and have ready any further items that may be required, e.g. swabs and sutures, without being asked. The care plan must be kept up to date. It is important to be aware at all times that the nurse is the patient's advocate. Counts are done as described above. The scrub nurse must be provided with all necessary dressings and bandages required for wound dressing. A check is then made for trauma; any noted must be documented.

Once the patient has left theatre the circulating nurse will clear all evidence of the last case from theatre and prepare for the next case.

Specimens

It is the circulating nurse's duty to label all specimens and forms correctly. She or he must check with the scrub nurse the exact nature of the specimen and ensure it is placed in the correct medium. The form will then be attached to the patient's notes for signature by the surgeon.

Health and Safety

Mention must be made of safeguards, not only for patients but also for practitioners. There are a number of inherent risks in the operating room, due to lifting and handling of patients and other heavy equipment, exposure to gases, hazardous substances, cytotoxic drugs, contaminated sharps and body fluids. The Control of Substances Hazardous to Health Regulations (Health and Safety Executive, 1992) cover all areas of concern in the operating theatre and document the appropriate measures to be taken.

Care of the patient undergoing surgery

Intra-operative care is the physical and psychological care given to the patient from the time of arrival in theatre until transfer to the recovery room. During this period the theatre practitioner must ensure that the patient fully understands what is happening at all times, to minimise anxiety.

The patient is collected from the ward by the theatre nurse, who may already have met the patient and discussed any problems or worries. As already mentioned, the emotional stress that is often experienced before an operation can be alleviated by a familiar face and a welcoming smile.

The theatre nurse must identify the patient by asking him or her to say his or her own name, then checking that the name and number of the patient's identification label corresponds with the medical and nursing notes.

It is the surgeon's duty to obtain the patient's permission to perform an operation. In obtaining consent the patient must also be informed of the nature of the operation, the benefits and the possible risks involved. It is the nurse's role to check that consent has been obtained and that the nature of the operation is clearly stated and legible. It is also the collecting nurse's responsibility to go through the pre-operative check list (see Figure 4.1) At this stage the theatre practitioner should also confirm that the patient has a responsible person collecting them who will be with them for 24 hours post-operatively.

	Yes	Comments
Identity band correct		
Correct notes		
Correct X-rays		
Consent form signed		
Operation site marked		
Operation site shaved		
Nil by mouth from		
Dentures removed		
Caps/crowns		
Jewellery and make-up removed		
Prosthesis identity		
Allergies		

Figure 4.1: Pre-operative checklist

Most new, purpose-built day units do not use anaesthetic rooms, but anaesthetise the patient in theatre. Patients are admitted to the ward and transferred to theatre on trolleys, which are also used as theatre tables. In some units patients are walked into theatre and transferred to a trolley post-operatively. The anaesthetising of patients in theatre minimises the number of times an unconscious patient has to be moved or transferred.

Unlike a regular theatre table, a day surgery trolley is modified to be used as a bed as well as a theatre table. It therefore has limitations: it is uncomfortable as a bed and has deficiencies as an operating table. Much thought and research has gone into the development of the day surgery trolley, but the problem of weight and manoeuvrability continues. However, despite its deficiencies, the ward/theatre trolley is more acceptable and efficient than transferring the patient between bed, operating table and bed again.

An operating table must incorporate many features which are also bed safety features, such as cot sides. But these sides can also cause a problem by getting in the way of the surgeon's legs during the operation, and they may make it difficult to reach the pedals for raising and lowering the table and changing the table position. The table must also be covered in non-slip anti-static materials, with anti-static wheels, to prevent patients slipping and the build-up of static electricity in an area where flammable gases and diathermy are used. It must have a solid braking system, be height adjustable and must be able to accommodate the positions necessary for all surgical specialties. The trolley must also be designed to accommodate any X-ray or image intensification equipment that may be required.

Accessories for the trolley include well padded arm supports, which should be placed at the elbow to prevent the arms from falling off the table, lithotomy poles, which must be placed at equal height and distance along the table; Lloyd Davies poles for a more comfortable way of placing patients in the lithotomy position for longer cases; varicose vein boards for abduction of legs in varicose vein surgery, which can also be used in the prone patient to accommodate the arms; and head rings for ENT and dental work. A selection of anti-static covered sandbags of various sizes help with positioning and Velcro straps hold patients safely in position. The prone mattress is designed to facilitate chest expansion in the prone position, it also follows the natural contours of the body in this position. Shoulder, ankle and heel pads can be used to prevent pressure on the legs and extend the neck for ENT surgery.

Once the patient has been anaesthetised and is unconscious he or she is totally dependent on the theatre team, who must ensure that all the patient's needs are met and that he or she comes to no harm. Therefore, the role of the nurse as the patient's advocate is critical in theatre. All staff working in theatre must be aware of potential hazards that can occur and actions that must be taken to prevent injury to the patient.

Positioning of the patient

Positioning a patient for an operative procedure is one of the most important duties of the circulating nurse. Patients who are anaesthetised cannot tell the nurse that they are uncomfortable from being improperly positioned. The unconscious patient who is positioned badly or carelessly is at risk of serious injury. Pressure created by rucked sheets can cause injury, especially in elderly patients, and nerve damage may occur as a result of over-enthusiastic positioning. All movements must be slowly and carefully performed, and if two limbs are involved there must be a nurse to position each one. Limbs must not be over-extended, they must always be in as normal a position as possible. Body alignment must be natural to prevent any muscle spasm. The head and neck must be particularly carefully aligned to prevent any neck damage. Nerve damage, especially to ulnar and brachial nerves, can be avoided by preventing pressure to specific areas. No part of the patients body must be in contact with metal to prevent burning from diathermy.

Correct positioning will provide easy access to the operation site for the surgeon, allow access for the anaesthetist and provide maximum safety for the patient. Patients must never be moved without prior consent from the anaesthetist. The anaesthetist will also be the person who will support the head during any positioning.

The positioning will depend on the type of surgery to be carried out, so the choice of position will be made by the surgeon. It is important that all members of the theatre staff are familiar with the operating table/trolley and accessories, such as armboards, head-rests and lithotomy poles (see Table 4.1).

Diathermy

Electrosurgery (diathermy) is potentially an extremely hazardous procedure. If carried out by untrained or careless staff it can cause horrific burns to the patient. Diathermy is used in most surgical operations where coagulation, to control haemorrhage or cutting of tissue, is required.

Table 4.1: Correct positioning of patients for surgery

Position	Surgery	Attachments	Method	Risks
Supine Patient flat on back	Abdominal and anything anteriorally	Arm rests; leg straps; heel supports	Good body alignment; feet not crossed; arms positioned anatomically and held securely to table	Calf pressure; nerve damage
Trendelenburg Head down supine position	Lower abdominal surgery, e.g. laparoscopy; varicose vein surgery	As above	As above; care not to over-tilt the table	As above; slipping off table
Reverse Trendelenburg Legs down supine position	Upper abdominal surgery; laparoscopic cholecystectomy	As above	As above	As above
Lithotomy Legs up in stirrups or Lloyd Davis supports	Gynae; GU; anal	Lithotomy poles with stirrups for ankle and instep; Lloyd Davis supports with Velcro straps	Patient positioned with buttocks over lower break in table; poles same height, legs supported; legs raised slowly and simultaneously; arms over chest or in armbands	Muscle strain; dislocation of hips; back strain; arms

Table 4.1: (contd)

Position	Surgery	Attachments	Method	Risks
Lateral Patient on side	Any that best exposes operation site	Back support; chest support; pillow between legs; Velcro straps	Patient turned to side; lower leg flexed; upper leg support; supports position; secured with straps	Patient falling; lower arm compression; knee pressure
Prone Patient on front	All operations on back, e.g. pilonidal sinus, varicose veins	Second trolley; prone mattress; pillow for legs	Patient rolled on to second prepared trolley at correct height; lower legs supported by pillows; arms positioned above head on extension board and secured	Falling; nerve damage to arms; airway obstruction necessitating quick return to supine

It is carried out by heating the tissues using high frequency electrosurgical current. The current is applied to the required point of contact via insulated forceps. Heat is produced as the cells resist the current causing coagulation and tissue destruction.

There are two basic types of circuits used in diathermy. In monopolar circuits the current is produced by the diathermy machine and conducted to a small active electrode, e.g. insulated forceps, which is brought into contact with the tissues. The current is conducted through the patient's body and is earthed via the patient plate into the machine. The patients plate consists of a salt-based gel, the best conductor, surrounded by an adhesive border. A metal strip protruding from the border takes the lead clamp that is connected to the diathermy machine.

In bipolar circuits coagulation occurs when the current is passed between the tips of the forceps and is not conducted through the patient's body. A patient plate is not, therefore, required.

Diathermy is activated by the surgeon by use of appropriate foot pedals or finger switches. The range of active electrodes used includes electrodes with a spatulated end, balls and buttons for coagulation, but these are not widely used in day surgery. Fine pointed ends and blades are used for cutting. Loop electrodes may be used in cervical areas in gynaecology. These must always be kept in a quiver when not in use to prevent accidental burning of the patient.

Dangers of diathermy

The greatest risk when using monopolar diathermy is a burn to the patient's skin. The cause of such burns is nearly always either the incorrect application of the patient plate or a break in the wire connecting the plate to the patient. Diathermy burns are also likely to occur when the patient's skin is in direct contact with solid metal. The current is diverted from earthing via the plate and is attracted to the metal, causing tissue destruction at the point of contact, which is where the current leaves the body.

Safeguards used during diathermy

Staff must be competent in their knowledge of how the diathermy machine operates and must know how to set it up correctly. Modern machines facilitate both mono and bipolar diathermy. All machines have built-in safety systems to prevent incorrect setting up. All lead inserts to the machine are of differing sizes so they cannot be wrongly inserted. Alarms will ring if the circuit is not complete.

The machine must be checked daily to ensure alarms are working. The patient plate must be checked to make sure it has not dried out. Careful consideration must be given to the positioning of the patient plate to ensure good contact is maintained. The plate is most effective when applied over a vascular muscular area. Fat is a poor conductor of electricity, and bony and hairy areas do not provide good contact. The skin must be intact and superfluous hair removed. There must not be any wrinkling of the plate.

The best place for the plate is the thigh. If this is not possible due to the nature of the operation other areas that can be used are the abdomen, buttocks, mid-back and lower back. The plate must be applied with the longest side closest to the operative site to attract the current and safely complete the circuit. The plate must remain dry and precautions should be taken to prevent pooling of flammable liquids in any cavity, under the body or on the plate itself.

Hypothermia

Although not a recognised problem area in day surgery because operating times are relatively short, the problem of heat loss should be taken into consideration when dealing with very young or very old patients. The theatre should be at an optimum temperature of between 19 and 23 °C. Heated gauze/material and heated mattresses may be used for infants.

Gynaecology

There are a number of gynaecological procedures that may be undertaken in the DSU.

Dilatation and curettage (D and C) involves dilatation of the cervix to allow access to the uterus and subsequent curettage of the endometrial lining. It is carried out on patients experiencing excessive menstrual bleeding or intra-menstrual bleeding, and for diagnostic purposes.

Termination of pregnancy is a similar procedure to a D and C, but with full suction evacuation from the uterus of all products of conception. Evacuation of retained products of conception (ERPC) may also be included in this area but remains a contentious issue as there is some discussion as to whether the DSU is suitable for emergency work. ERPC is carried out on the authors' unit and provides a faster and more effective service for patients who might otherwise have to wait a long time in the accident and emergency department for a bed, then be admitted to a ward where they may have to wait until the end of an operating list before the procedure can be carried out.

Diathermy to vulval warts and abnormal cervical cells is done to effect destruction. Bartholin's cysts are drained and marsupialised.

Hysteroscopy is the expansion of the uterus with saline or carbon dioxide (CO_2) to allow the introduction of a telescope to view the endometrium of the uterus, and to allow a biopsy to be taken for diagnostic purposes.

Laparoscopy entails inflating the abdominal cavity with CO_2 to allow the safe passage of a telescope into the abdomen. This procedure is used for diagnostic purposes, e.g. to diagnose endometriosis, ovarian abnormalities and to test patency of Fallopian tubes. It is also used for diathermy to the ovaries and endometriosis. To test the patency of the Fallopian tubes a dye is introduced via the cervix and, if the tubes are functioning normally, can be seen escaping the fimbriated end of the tubes. Laparoscopic sterilisation requires the attachment of clips to the Fallopian tubes to obstruct patency.

Laparoscopic surgery

Laparoscopic surgery, also known as minimal access surgery (MAS) or keyhole surgery, is becoming increasingly popular for day cases because it decreases tissue trauma and increases efficiency. The confirmed benefits of MAS are reduced post-operative pain, accelerated recovery, lower incidence of post-operative respiratory complications, early return to full activity or work, and significant reductions in wound-related complications (Cuschieri, 1993).

The theatre nurse must be competent in the care and use of the complex equipment required for this type of surgery, she or he must know how it all works and how to deal with any complications that may arise, and should be familiar with the hazards that may occur.

This section pertains to both gynaecological and general surgery.

Specialist equipment in laparoscopic surgery

Insufflator – used to introduce CO_2 into the abdominal cavity at a safe rate to ensure good views and enable the operator to safely introduce the laparoscope.

Pneumoperitoneal (Verres) needle – the gas is introduced via this needle normally at the lower border of the umbilicus.

CO_2 is used as it is the gas most easily absorbed by the body and it is non-combustible. It is soluble, which lessens the risk of air embolism if it is accidentally introduced into a blood vessel.

Trocar and **cannulae** are inserted through various small incisions in the abdomen to allow the introduction of instrumentation.

Telescopes are always fibre-optic and must be handled carefully. They may have differing angles but are generally 0°. They require a fibre-optic light lead and light source. All modern telescopes are now autoclavable. Care must be taken with the cleaning of scopes and leads. This should be done under warm running water with detergent to remove all debris, taking special care of lenses.

The camera, if used on the end of the telescope, must be of a special high resolution type and a sterile camera drape must be used to prevent contamination of the operation site. All equipment must be carefully checked and inspected before use by a competent member of the theatre team to ensure patient safety and efficient use of theatre time.

Hazards of laparoscopy

Table 4.2 outlines the major complications that can occur during laparoscopic surgery.

Extra equipment required includes suction equipment, diathermy capability, a method of ligating the blood vessels, ducts and tubes, and special forceps for grasping and dissection. In all laparoscopic procedures a set of abdominal instruments should always be available to perform open laparotomy in an emergency.

General surgery

A large percentage of day surgery work is performed under a local anaesthetic. Although the removal of 'lumps and bumps' may be minor to theatre staff, it can cause great anxiety to the patient. No surgery is minor to the patient.

The local anaesthetic patient should be checked, taken to the theatre and cared for, and returned to the ward/day room area by the same person. If the nurse can quickly develop a rapport with the patient, this can considerably reduce anxiety. Careful explanation of events and giving post-operative information will further assist in the patient's compliance.

Table 4.2: Major complications of laparoscopic surgery

Potential hazard	Causes	Nursing action	Outcome
Haemorrhage due to severing of major vessels	Inserting trocars without direct vision; poor surgical technique	Be prepared for laparotomy	Efficient transition to open laparotomy without compromising patient safety
Gas embolism	Vessels may be punctured while going into peritoneum and CO_2 enters the bloodstream	Adequate monitoring: ECG, pulse oximetry, capnograph monitor. Ensure all CO_2 removed	Minimise hazards; detection of complications
Regurgitation of stomach contents	Raising of intra-abdominal pressure causing pressure on the stomach	Nasogastric tube passed by anaesthetist	Minimise hazards and early detection of complications
Pneumothorax	Pneumoperitoneum may cause pressure and rupture the pleura	Check for cardiac arrythmias, tachycardia and hypotension	Turn off insufflator; change patient position to supine; chest drain available
Subcutaneous emphysema	Over insufflation of abdomen, incorrect position of insufflating needle	Turn off insufflator; correct monitoring of insufflator	

Laparoscopic surgery

Research has shown that, at present, the only laparoscopic operation acceptable as standard in general surgery is cholecystectomy (Cuschieri, 1993), although laparoscopic inguinal hernia repair and laparoscopic appendicectomy are regularly performed in some centres. In the authors' unit laparoscopic cervical sympathectomy has been carried out. Chest drainage equipment must be to hand for this procedure.

Hernias

There are four hernias that can be repaired/reduced as day-case procedures: inguinal, femoral, umbilical and small incisional.

The technique used to repair a hernia will depend on the surgeon's preference, but the types of materials and the methods used must be known to the nurse. These include non-absorbable darns, two layer repairs (Shouldice), the use of mesh and laparoscopic repair, if undertaken.

If a patient is not suitable for a general anaesthetic or if the patient prefers, he may have a hernia repair under local anaesthetic. If this is to be carried out it is important that the patient is properly assessed by a consultant in the out-patient department. Some hernia repairs may not be suitable for LA repair, e.g. repair of recurrent hernias.

As with all LA procedures carried out in theatre the nurse must be especially aware of the patient's needs and anxieties. A nurse or member of the theatre team must sit with the patient at all times throughout the procedure, explaining in simple non-technical terms exactly what is happening and repeating the surgeon's instructions if necessary. The nurse should also explain that the patient will feel pressure but should not feel pain; if they do feel pain more LA can be given. Intravenous sedation may be used. In the authors' unit Medazolam is the drug of choice. This can facilitate patient compliance and helps reduce anxiety.

It is very easy for the scrub nurse and surgeon to forget that the patient is awake. Patients do not want to hear the gory details of their surgery, therefore, it is important that the scrub nurse knows the procedure so she is able to follow the surgeon. The surgeon should be discouraged from saying 'knife' loudly, as this may terrify the patient. The use of diathermy should be explained to the patient before the procedure starts.

Varicose veins

The methods in use for surgical treatment of varicose veins are high tie of the long saphenous vein and stripping of the long saphenous vein, either to the knee or, if possible, the ankle, both of which may also require multiple avulsions of minor perforations of valves that show incompetence.

The operation is performed in the Trendelenburg position, to aid venous return, with the legs abducted. It may be complicated by a need to reposition the patient from supine to prone to operate on the backs of the legs. This will require redraping after repositioning. A supportive bandage or stocking is applied at the finish of the operation.

Anal surgery

Anal surgery requires the patient to be in the lithotomy position. Sigmoidoscopy or proctoscopy is often undertaken before anal surgery to confirm diagnosis and should always be available.

An anal fissure is a small crack in the lining of the skin of the anus caused by trauma from a tight anal sphincter. A small incision is made in the anal sphincter muscle – sphincterotomy – or an anal stretch may be performed.

Polyps occur in the lower rectum and are removed after inserting a dissolvable suture through their base to prevent bleeding or by the use of diathermy. Anal warts and tags may be diathermied or excised. An anal fistula is a small tunnel through the tissues between the skin and the rectum. This is treated by cutting the skin down to the rectum and laying the fistula open.

Small haemorrhoids may be treated by injection of a sclerosing agent, e.g. phenol, or by dissection and ligation before surgical removal.

The dressings used for all of the above are normally paraffin gauze, padding and 'T' bandage.

Breast lumps

Removal of small breast lumps and breast biopsy are usually carried out under general anaesthetic, but occasionally small lumps may be removed under a local anaesthetic.

If a breast lump is thought to be malignant, a wider area around the lump may be excised. In general, a large wound that would necessitate wound drainage is not suitable for day-case surgery, although in occasional circumstances a fine vacuum drain will be inserted for removal 24 hours later by the community nurse.

The purpose of wound drainage is the removal of air and fluid from a cavity to the body surface, where the fluid soaks into a dressing or is directed into a closed vacuumed container.

There are many other small operative procedures carried out in the day unit. It is impossible to describe them all, but the theatre nurse must check the list and be aware of any extra instrumentation that may be required for specific cases. For example, operations such as tongue tie release or oral procedures must have mouth gags available.

Orthopaedic surgery

As with all specialties there is an increase in the use of day surgery in orthopaedics. There are a number of appropriate operations included in the Royal College of Surgeons *Guidelines* (1992).

Excision of ganglion. A ganglion is the commonest cystic swelling. It is most often found on the back of the wrist but can also be found on other joints such as fingers and ankle.

Decompression of carpal tunnel. Carpal tunnel syndrome is the constriction of the median nerve, which causes discomfort in the hand. Treatment involves dividing the sheath to decompress the nerve.

Dupytren's contracture is the flexion contracture of one or more of the fingers from thickening and shortening of the palma facia. Surgery entails excision of the thickened part of the palma facia.

Trigger finger occurs when the thickening and construction of the mouth of a fibrous digital sheath interferes with the free gliding of the tendons. Treatment is by incising the fibrous sheath.

Ingrowing toe-nail operations and all the above procedures may be carried out under a general anaesthetic, local anaesthetic or regional block. Factors contributing to the choice of anaesthetic include the size of the operation, the surgeon's choice and, of course, the patient's preference, which will depend on how anxious he or she is.

Other operations appropriate for day surgery are manipulation and injection of steroids to joints, removal of pins, plates or screws, amputation of the fingers and lesser toes, and arthroscopy.

Arthroscopy can be carried out on most joints, e.g. knee, shoulder, wrist, ankle, hip and spine, but it is most commonly performed on the knee joint. An arthroscopy is the direct inspection of the interior of a joint. The operation is carried out under tourniquet with continuous irrigation. A fine 30° telescope is introduced through a cannula and the joint cavity is filled with saline to allow good vision. Arthroscopies are carried out for diagnosis of knee complaints and also for trimming of meniscal tears, removal of loose bodies and reconstruction of cruciate ligament damage. The care of arthroscopic equipment is the same as that described for laparoscopic equipment.

Other orthopaedic operations that are being increasingly carried out on the DSU are open reduction and internal fixation of fractures. This facilitates the use of image intensification and the application of plaster casts, which should be readily available.

In the authors' unit shoulder arthroscopy is carried out for diagnosis and treatment of common conditions such as impingement syndrome and repair of dislocated shoulders. These procedures can be carried out arthroscopically or by proceeding to open operation.

Many orthopaedic operations are carried out in a bloodless field under pneumatic tourniquet. The pneumatic cuff is inflated with a non-flammable gas to raise the pressure. A correctly applied tourniquet cuff should compress the vessels just sufficiently to stop arterial blood flow and no more. The limb is elevated before the cuff is inflated, to allow the blood to drain from the vessels. The peripheral vessels can then be emptied by the use of a rubber Esmarchs bandage tightly wound round the drained limb or a Rhys-Davies exsanguinator.

Special care must be taken when a patient is having the operation under LA as the tourniquet is often the most uncomfortable part of the procedure.

The tourniquet is never released until the surgeon gives instructions for deflation. A check is made before the patient leaves the operating theatre to confirm that the tourniquet has been removed and that the circulation is satisfactory. The maximum recommended time for tourniquet is 2 hours. Tourniquet times must be documented.

The following safety aspects must be considered when applying a tourniquet:-

- it must be situated away from joints and areas of broken skin;
- an appropriate size of cuff must be used;
- adequate padding must be used;
- rings must be removed from the fingers of the operation arm;
- the solution used to prep the skin should not be allowed to run under the cuff, as it could cause a chemical burn;
- time of commencement must be noted;
- notes must be checked to make sure that the patient has not had arterial surgery and does not have an existing deep vein thrombosis;

- check that it is being applied to the correct limb;
- readings must be correct to compress vessels but not induce ischaemia, i.e. thigh: double the patient's systolic blood pressure; arm: 50 mm Hg above the patient's systolic blood pressure.

ENT surgery

The scope of work that can be carried out by the ENT surgeon is constantly under debate. The simple aural procedures, such as examination under microscope, clearing of the external canal, polyp removal and myringotomies, with insertion of either short- or long-term tubes, are well within the range of day surgery.

Myringotomy is the perforation of the ear drum to clear the middle ear of 'glue'. To keep the incision open, a small tube called a grommet is inserted. This also equalises the pressure between the external and middle ear, so improving hearing. Myringoplasty is the replacment of part or all of the tympanic membrane with a fat or haemogenous muscle graft. For a fat graft a small incision is made in the ear lobe, fat removed and replaced in the tympanic defect. For a muscle graft a posterior ear incision is made and muscle removed before proceeding to myringoplasty through this external incision. Tympanoplasty is where the operation is extended to include reconstruction of ossicles to restore hearing.

The ENT surgeons at the authors' unit are visiting consultants and have no beds in the hospital, therefore, any patients with problems have to be transported to another centre. For this reason adenoidectomy and tonsillectomy (Ts and As) patients are carefully assessed by consultants and nurses before being placed on the waiting list. They are all operated on in the morning and stay in the unit well into the afternoon to observe for problems of primary haemorrhage. In the basket of procedures recommended by the Royal College of Surgeons Ts and As were considered unlikely to be performed safely on a day-care basis. Adenoidectomy, by its physiology, is only performed on children.

When dealing with Ts and As extra care must be taken in the intra- and post-operative periods as this procedure carries a small, but real, danger. Bipolar diathermy is increasingly used to control bleeding of the tonsil beds, but ties of choice should always be available. Any procedure that can embarrass respiration with a potential to cause oedema of the throat presents a further threat to patient safety.

Operations on the throat and nose may also cause ingestion of blood and irritation of the stomach, causing nausea and vomiting. Intra-operatively some nasal patients may have throat packs to prevent this.

Nasal procedures that produce little or no bleeding, such as washouts, antrostomies, sub-mucosal diathermy and diathermy to Littles area, are well within day surgery recommendations, as are minor surgery to the lips, tongue, salivary glands and small palate biopsies. More complex surgery with increased haemorrhage potential, such as nasal polypectomy, turbinectomy and sub-mucosal resection, require careful selection. In the authors' unit any nasal packs inserted are removed by the surgeon before discharge and, as with Ts and As, patients remain longer in the unit.

Surgery to the nose may be preceded by the application of 5 per cent cocaine paste to assist in vasoconstriction and local anaesthesia. Moffat's solution, a mixture of sodium bicarbonate, liquid cocaine and 1 in 1000 topical adrenalin, may also be used to pack the nose pre-operatively. Citanest, a solution of pilocarpine and 1 in 200 000 adrenalin, can be injected sub-mucosally to achieve the same effect.

Procedures on the throat, such as rigid laryngoscopy and micro-laryngoscopy, are performed to diagnose and treat abnormalities. A microscope may be used, and the lens must be one of lower resolution than that used for the ears. An extended head position with a shoulder support is adopted.

Bronchoscopy may be performed with a rigid bronchoscope, but more usually a flexible scope is used. All specialist equipment, e.g. long suction catheters and forceps, should be available.

Specialist equipment

The range of specialist equipment used in ENT surgery includes: head rings for immobilisation during nose and ear operations; microscopes, which must be carefully positioned with the various arms manoeuvrable and with sterile covers; ENT headlights that provide a direct beam of light from a harness on the surgeon's head; lighted nasal speculae are also available. Suction must be available for all ENT cases.

Urology

This area may cross over into general surgery. Both undertake:

•   circumcisions – removal of the foreskin of the penis;

- excision of epididymal cysts – cysts in the tissue surrounding the scrotum;
- orchidopexy – placement of an undescended testicle into the scrotal sac;
- orchidectomy – removal of one or both testes due to adult undescended testicle, trauma or tumours. This procedure may also include the replacement with a testicular prosthesis;
- surgical treatment of varicocele – ligation of testicular varicose veins;
- surgical treatment of hydrocele – a collection of fluid between the layers covering the testicle (tunica vaginalis) requiring removal of fluid and sac;
- vasectomies – division of the vas deferens bilaterally to cause sterility. This may be undertaken using general or local anaesthetic;
- reversal of vasectomy – an attempt to reconnect the vas deferens to restore fertility.

Cystoscopy

Cystoscopy is often used in urology. The cystoscope may be flexible, with integral fibre-optic telescope, a connection to allow filling of the bladder with normal saline to facilitate vision and a second channel to allow for fine biopsy or grasping forceps to be used. Flexible cystoscopy is often performed under local anaesthetic, e.g. Instillagel, or solely with KY jelly or a similar lubricant. All scopes must be well lubricated to prevent urethral trauma.

If a flexiscope is used under a general anaesthetic the patient's bladder should always be emptied using a disposable catheter as the scope has no emptying facility.

Rigid cystoscopes consist of a sheath and obturator to enter the bladder. The obturator is then withdrawn and a telescope with a bridge inserted. The scope has a connection for normal saline to inflate the bladder and a light lead attachment. Depending on the type and make of scope there may be further channels for the introduction of forceps, ureteric catheters and diathermy electrodes. Otherwise a catheter slide can be used.

In male patients the urethra will be inspected under direct vision using a 0° telescope. Strictures can be dilated or slit using a uretherotome. The telescope is then changed for the more common 30° or 70° angle. Small bladder biopsies can be taken or bladder stones or small tumours removed. A ureteroscope can be advanced into either of the ureters under direct vision and small calculi (stones) can be either crushed with a lithotripter or removed using a dormia basket. A double 'J' stent may then be inserted from the kidney pelvis to the bladder to keep the ureter patent – this may be removed at a later date either with a flexi or rigid scope and grasping forceps.

Ureteric catheterisation may be performed and the scope removed, leaving the catheters in situ for diagnostic retrograde pyelograms to be undertaken.

Small recurrent bladder tumours or small prostate gland regrowths can be excised by performing a trans-urethral resection (TUR). The resectoscope has the facility to slice through the prostate with loop cutting diathermy, bleeding can then be controlled using coagulation diathermy. The bladder is irrigated for TUR with glycine solution to prevent bladder burns, and must be well irrigated throughout the procedure to maintain good visualisation. The bladder may be gently syringed at the end of the procedure to remove debris. This debris is often put through a sieve to isolate a specimen for histology. TUR requires a patient plate and a cutting and coagulating capacity; the setting will be at the surgeon's discretion. All safety measures and precautions must be observed.

Only small resections are suitable for day surgery because of the risk of haemorrhage and the need for continuous irrigation in larger cases. Any solutions used must be checked by two nurses and the bladder must not be allowed to empty as this would cause air to enter the system. A supply of various bladder catheters, syringes and water for inflating the catheter balloon, ureteric catheters, guide wires, measuring jugs and spigots should be available.

Many urology patients with bladder tumours have cytotoxic drugs instilled into the bladder to provide direct tumour contact. The patient is catheterised, the bladder emptied and the drug introduced. The patient then turns on his or her back, right side, front and left side for 30 minutes each. Great care must be taken by the practitioner when using or preparing these drugs as they can themselves be carcinogenic.

Gloves, aprons and long sleeved gowns should be worn and the eyes protected with goggles. The patient normally has six treatments at intervals prescribed by the surgeon, anything from weekly to monthly.

Oral and maxillofacial surgery

Oral and maxillofacial surgery covers all aspects of dental work under general anaesthetic. This may be the removal of first teeth in children or permanent removal in adults. Other operations may include apicectomy (retrograde root filling) following removal of root cysts.

A full set of dental forceps for upper and lower teeth must be available. The upper extraction forceps are always straight and the lower are angled. The heads of the forceps are of differing widths to facilitate removal of differing teeth and are beaked for a firmer grip.

Deciduous teeth are nominated by letter starting at the front with two 'A's. Adult permanent teeth are nominated by number (see Figure 4.2). The most common operation is the extraction of impacted '8's, or wisdom teeth. This is performed by incising along the gum margin, exposing the bone and creating a window in the bone to allow dental instruments to elevate the tooth out from below. Either a dental chisel and mallet are used to create the window or a dental drill with various burrs. Other specialised instrumentation includes mouth gags and props, tongue and cheek extractors, periosteal elevators and dental elevators. The gum flap is sutured back with an absorbable suture material. Local anaesthetic can be injected peri-operatively to aid haemostatis as well as providing post-operative pain relief. All teeth must be examined to ensure complete removal of roots.

To perform an apicectomy dental amalgam must be available and an amalgam gun to deliver the amalgam to the tooth root.

Deciduous

    R   EDCBA ABCDE   L

_____

    R   EDCBA ABCDE   L

Adult

    R   87654321 12345678   L

_____

    R   87654321 12345678   L

Figure 4.2: Nomination of deciduous and adult permanent teeth

Suction must always be available and throat packs are always inserted by the anaesthetist pre-operatively. It is the nurses duty to inform the anaesthetist that this pack has been removed at the end of the case. Dental packs with an integral tie attached, usually wet, are placed over the operation site to provide pressure. A heavy horseshoe shaped head ring is used to stabilise the head during the operation.

References

American Operating Room Nurse (1987) Recommended practice for pre-operative skin prep. AORN Journal 46(4): 719–724.

Carrington A (1991) Theatre nursing as a profession. British Jounal of Theatre Nursing April 1(1): 5–7.

Cucshieri MA (1993) Minimal Access Surgery Implications for the NHS. London: HMSO.

Freshwater D (1992) Pre-operative preparation of skin – a review of the literature. Surgical Nurse 5(5): 6–10.

Hayward J (1975) Information – A Prescription Against Pain. London: Royal College of Nursing.

Health and Safety Executives (1988) Control of Substances Hazardous to Health Regulations. London: HMSO.

McGee P (1992) Theatre nurses face elimination. British Journal of Nursing 1(11): 535–536.

NHS Management Executive (1993) Day Surgery Task Force Report. London: HMSO.

Nightingale K (1986) Is theatre nursing in jeopardy? NATNEWS 23(6): 18–19.

Penn S (1993) Education in day surgery. A nursing view. Journal of One Day Surgery Autumn 3(2): 10–11.

Royal College of Surgeons (1992) Commission on the Provision of Surgical Services. Guidelines for Day Case Surgery. London: RCS.

Sutherland R (1994) Is this the way forward? British Journal of Theatre Nursing 4(1): 12–13.

Wicker P (1987) The role of the theatre nurse. Senior Nurse 7(4): 19–21.

Further reading

Adams A (1990) Theatre Nursing. London: Heinemann Nursing.

Adams J, Hamblen D (1990) Outline of Orthopaedics. London: Churchill Livingstone.

Anderton JM, Keen RI, Neare R (1988) Positioning the Surgical Patient. London: Butterworth.

Blackburn E (1994) Prevention of hypothermia during anaesthesia. British Journal Theatre Nursing 4(8): 9–14.

Brigden RJ (1988) Operating Table Technique, 5th edn. London: Churchill Livingstone.

Bull PD (1991) Lecture Notes on Diseases of the Ear, Nose and Throat, 7th edn. Oxford: Blackwell Scientific Publications.

Ethicon (1980) A Digest of Obstetrical and Gynaecological Procedures. Edinburgh: Ethicon.

Ethicon (1993) Suture Material and Surgical Needles. Edinburgh: Ethicon.

James J (1984) Handbook of Urology. Lippincott Nursing Series London: Harper and Row.

McHale J, Tingle J (1995) Consent to treatment. British Journal Nursing 4(4): 239.

National Association of Theatre Nurses (1988) Theatre Safeguards. Harrogate: NATN.

National Association of Theatre Nurses (1989) Principles of Safe Practice in the Operating Theatre. Harrogate: NATN.

Oakley K (1990) X-ray precautions. Nursing Times 88(6): 50–51.

Oakley K (1994) Making sense of universal precautions. Nursing Times 90(27): 35–36.

Warren M (1983) Operating Theatre Nursing. Lippincott Nursing Series. London: Harper and Row.

Wells R (1986) The great conspiracy – informed consent. Nursing Times 82(21): 22–25.

Wicker P (1992) Making sense of electrosurgery. Nursing Times 88(45): 31–33.

Chapter 5
Recovery nursing in day surgery

Dawn Wotton

Introduction

This chapter describes the role of the recovery nurse in day surgery, and the ideal recovery room. It discusses the need for the patient to recover from anaesthesia sufficiently well to be discharged a few hours later, and explores the ways in which the nurse facilitates this. The analgesics in common use are described, with their advantages and disadvantages, and the use of opiate analgesia is also discussed. The chapter looks at the risks to the patient during the immediate post-operative phase and describes the necessary action by the nurse should emergencies occur. The essential equipment required in all recovery rooms is described, and the skills required of a recovery nurse and ways in which standards of care may be monitored are also discussed.

Day surgery recovery room staff requirements and duties are similar to those of any recovery room. In most cases, one nurse can comfortably look after three self-ventilating patients. The recovery area should be as close as possible to the operating theatre where surgery is performed, and the equipment, monitoring, supervision and management must be equivalent to those in a normal recovery area. Written protocols should cover admission and discharge, routines for checking equipment and drugs, establishing the duties of all medical, nursing and paramedical staff, problems and how to handle them, and lines of communication.

Before setting up a new recovery room, it is advisable to visit as many others as possible to find out the good and bad features.

The recovery area needs to be open and uncluttered with no structural obstructions. Every trolley bay should be visible from anywhere in the room, and there should be an 'emergency area' where the defibrillator and all the equipment for managing a cardiac arrest are kept. This should be easily accessible from all trolley bays. It will need its own power outlets for keeping the batteries that run the portable equipment charged.

Each trolley bay will need its own service utilities on the wall at the head of the trolley. Ideally there should be:

- high pressure oxygen wall outlets equipped with flow-meters;
- high-flow suction outlets, including receiver, tubing, sucker and a range of suction catheters;
- electric power outlets;
- spotlights;
- shelves.

All the recovery room bays should be identical. Emergency power is essential in case the main supply fails; this will automatically switch on if there is a power failure. There should be a non-slip floor. Walls and ceilings should be light, neutral colours because stronger colours may reflect on the patient's skin causing confusion about his or her colour. There should be a hand basin with a liquid soap dispenser and paper towel holder.

Each bay needs its own pulse oximeter. These devices enable blood oxygen saturation to be measured via a small probe that fits on a fingertip. This is probably the single most useful monitoring device in the recovery area.

There should be an emergency trolley containing the drugs and equipment necessary for dealing with emergency resuscitation and cardiac arrests, and mechanical ventilation equipment should also be at hand.

There should be some means of screening for each patient, and an emergency call bell should be situated in each recovery bay.

Each recovery bay should store:

- oxygen masks and tubing;
- T-pieces for delivering oxygen to patients with endotracheal tubes or laryngeal masks;
- suction catheters and tubing;
- oropharyngeal airways;
- self-inflating breathing bags;

- black face-masks;
- vomit bowls;
- bandages and tape;
- sphygmomanometer and stethoscope.

There should also be emergency trays and trolleys for cardiac arrest, re-intubation, anaphylaxis and malignant hyperthermia.

It should be routine to check all equipment before receiving a patient. Fatalities can occur for lack of something simple like proper suction tubing or because of a disconnected oxygen line.

At the beginning of each shift the recovery nurse should ensure that the resuscitation trolley has been checked and signed for in the maintenance book, disposable items have been replaced, sharps and rubbish containers are clean and empty, oxygen and suction supplies are adequate, suction canisters and tubing are clean and working and the alarm system is working, and that nothing is out of date.

Before each patient arrives it is the nurse's duty and responsibility to check that an oxygen mask is connected and ready, the suction is switched on and working, the pulse oximeter is switched on and working, and an ambu or re-breathing bag is available.

Before being transported any distance from theatre, the patient should have a stable cardiovascular system and be breathing adequately. The anaesthetic handover should include the name and age of the patient, significant medical conditions, procedure performed, details of vital signs, details of any incidents that occurred during surgery, analgesia given and anticipated needs, the patient's anxiety level, monitoring and investigation required. The anaesthetist should also tell the nursing staff where he or she will be so that rapid contact can be made if the need arises. The anaesthetist should not be far away while the patient is still in the recovery area.

The anaesthetist is responsible for supervising the recovery period, accompanying the patient to the recovery room, the handover to the nursing staff, providing written and verbal instructions to the recovery room staff, specifying requirements for the patient and remaining close by until the patient is safe to leave in the care of the nursing staff. The surgeon is responsible for authorising the discharge of a patient from the recovery room when it depends on a surgical decision and being available to consult with the anaesthetist about the patient's welfare.

The post-anaesthetic assessment is usually the responsibility of the anaesthetist.

The nursing staff handover to the ward should include details of special nursing requirements, such as position of the patient, precautions about dressings, nursing, notes, charts and X-rays as appropriate.

Perceptions of the recovery room

If the patient is still under the influence of the anaesthetic, the airway will need support and the pharynx and mouth must be clear of secretions. At this stage the patient may not respond to any stimuli. Plantar reflexes may not react or, if the patient is lightening, will show an upgoing response. The pupils may not react to light. As the patient lightens, gaze becomes divergent and the pupils constrict in reaction to light. A few moments before awakening, the pupils dilate and the patient may start to move his or her limbs, and to shiver. The pulse and blood pressure often rise. The patient may then take a breath and sigh just before opening his or her eyes.

Hearing is the first sense to return. Voices, to the patient, are very loud, distorted and sometimes frightening. Light may seem unduly bright and hurt the eyes. Vision is blurred, arms and legs feel heavy, and pain may be severe. Finally, sense of locality and memory return. The patient may feel giddy and disorientated.

Initial assessment

On admission to the recovery room, the following should be checked in the order given.

Airway

Make sure that the patient has a clear airway, is breathing, and that the air is moving freely in and out of the chest.

If necessary, gently suck out the patient's mouth and pharynx . If the patient is still unconscious, make sure the airway is supported, inserting an oral airway if necessary. Administer oxygen and attach a pulse oximeter.

Breathing

Check that the patient's chest is moving and air can be felt flowing in and out of the mouth. Look for any signs of cyanosis and note the reading on the pulse oximeter.

Circulation

Once the patient's airway and breathing have been checked, measure the blood pressure, pulse rate and rhythm, note the perfusion status and record.

Length of stay

In day surgery the length of stay in the recovery room is usually minimal. Patients wake quickly and return to the ward area almost immediately. In the author's unit, 10 minutes is the average length of stay.

The minimum criteria for discharge to the ward are:

- stable heart rate and blood pressure;
- satisfactory oxygen saturation on room air;
- a conscious patient able to lift his or her head from the pillow on command;
- a pain-free patient;
- no excessive loss from drains or bleeding from wound sites;
- completed observation charts.

Before sending the patient back to the ward the recovery nurse should remove all unnecessary intravenous lines and the electrocardiogram electrodes. She or he should also check that the medical and nursing staff have completed all notes and charts and send them back to the ward with the patient. Clear and concise notes on the patient's state in the recovery room will help the ward staff to identify any deterioration quickly. A nurse should always accompany the patient back to the ward.

Before a patient is discharged home, he or she should be awake and fully orientated, have no surgical complications or anaesthetic complications, such as dizziness or nausea, no unsteadiness on standing, no uncontrolled pain or breathing problems, and vital signs should be stable.

For the first 24 hours following general anaesthesia patients must be told not to drive a motor vehicle, use machinery that requires judgement or skill, drink alcohol, cook, sign any legal documents, or be the only person in charge of children or other dependants. They should also be advised not to lock doors behind them.

Studies show that despite these warnings, nearly 10 per cent of day surgery patients who have undergone a general anaesthetic drive themselves home. It is difficult to evaluate the extent of recovery following general anaesthesia. No single test can accurately demonstrate whether a patient is free from the effects of anaesthesia and is safe to leave hospital.

In the author's unit the discharge procedure is that patients are escorted by a competent adult. They have written instructions describing what they are to do when they reach home. These are detailed, describing the medication they are to take, what the effects of the procedure are likely to be and what to do if any problems arise. They need to have access to a telephone at home and they have the telephone numbers of the day unit and hospital. The unit also offers a 24-hour enquiry facility via a mobile telephone carried by senior staff out of hours. Patients have a follow-up appointment as necessary.

General anaesthesia should be reduced in the afternoons allowing sufficient time for patients to recover fully before discharge.

Adverse effects of pain in the recovery room

Pain is the most common cause of patient suffering in the recovery room. Although it is easy to control, this responsibility is often delegated to the most inexperienced member of the surgical team. A nonchalant attitude to pain control is inexcusable.

Pain causes restlessness and excitability, which increases oxygen consumption and may lead to hypoxia. It contributes to post-operative nausea and vomiting, and causes the blood pressure to rise. Hypertension makes the heart work harder and may precipitate myocardial ischaemia. Pain decreases hepatic and renal blood flow, delaying the metabolism and excretion of drugs. It prevents the patient from deep breathing, and if it is painful to move about, the patient will lie still and blood will flow more slowly, especially through the limbs. This predisposes to deep vein thrombosis and pulmonary embolism. Uncontrolled pain increases the chance of infection and wound breakdown.

The type of operation, site of incision and individual variation determine the severity of pain. Individuals vary in their response to pain and also in their response to analgesics. There are often complex psychosocial factors involved. Different ethnic groups respond in different ways to pain and their expectations and tolerance vary widely. Older people often do not report as much pain as younger people. However, whenever a patient complains of pain it must be treated and not ignored.

Pain is less likely to be distressing if it is expected or if the patient knows that it will only be temporary. It may help if the patient knows why he is in pain and is not anxious about the outcome of the surgery, therefore, communication with patients prior to surgery is important. This can prove difficult in the day surgery setting as patients are admitted only a short time before surgery itself and the time spent with each patient is minimal, and heightens the importance of concise information-giving.

Staff attitude can be a contributory factor to pain control. Control will be poor if staff consider pain to be 'psychological'. Pain control measures in the recovery room must work quickly to reduce harmful stress and must be designed to meet each individual's needs.

The use of analgesia in recovery

Every recovery room needs a reference book on drugs. This should include a formulary such as the *British National Formulary*, which is jointly published by the British Medical Association and the Royal Pharmaceutical Society of Great Britain. It is essential to have a drug interaction and compatibility guide. Many drugs are chemically incompatible with each other. If in any doubt, check with the hospital pharmacist first.

Despite the expansion of day surgery, the percentage of operations performed on a day basis is limited by the effectiveness of post-operative pain control. Local anaesthetics may provide excellent supplementary analgesia during the post-operative period.

Non-steroidal anti-inflammatory drugs

Non-steroidal anti-inflammatory drugs (NSAIDs) are commonly used in day surgery. Drugs used include diclofenac and ketorolac. They do not cause respiratory depression. However, these agents are contraindicated in asthma, peptic ulceration and renal impairment. They affect platelet function and their use, theoretically, leads to increased bleeding, but this risk may be clinically insignificant. NSAIDs produce few cardiorespiratory effects. They can also reduce opioid requirement and emesis, and, therefore, unplanned hospital admissions. Controversy will continue to surround these drugs for the reasons described in Chapter 3, and whether their adverse effects will prevent their widespread use in day surgery remains to be seen.

Opioids

The term 'opioid' describes a substance that binds to opioid receptors, and is commonly used to denote opiate and narcotic analgesics. Opioids produce analgesia, a reduction in metabolic and autonomic response to surgery and a reduction in the amount of anaesthetic required.

Fentanyl is a popular supplement to inhalation anaesthesia. At usual doses, its peak analgesic action takes approximately four minutes and its duration of analgesia is 30 minutes. Fentanyl is 10 times more potent than morphine and prolonged respiratory depression may occur.

Alfentanil is a synthetic opioid with an analgesic potency four times that of morphine and a duration of action one third that of fentanyl. Its short duration of action makes it particularly suitable for day-case anaesthesia and it may be given intermittently (IV) or by infusion.

Anaesthetics used in day-case surgery

Intravenous agents

A rapid return to fitness is important after day surgery. Anaesthetists will, therefore, wish to use induction agents with a rapid anaesthetic action, pain-free injection, no involuntary movements and rapid recovery. Of the commonly-used intravenous induction agents available, propofol and thiopentone produce good induction and recovery results.

Inhalational agents

Halothane, enflurane and isoflurane are still popular agents for day surgery. Sevoflurane and desflurane, although not currently available in all markets, deserve mention.

Total intravenous anaesthesia (TIVA)

Maintenance of anaesthesia may be achieved using TIVA with propofol and alfentanil. This anaesthetic regimen, coupled with spontaneous respiration of oxygen, provides stable anaesthesia with minimum post-operative morbidity. If it is necessary to ventilate the patient, TIVA may still be used for maintenance of anaesthesia.

The additional drug costs involved in TIVA are insignificant when unit overheads, theatre disposables and staff salaries are included in costing an anaesthetic technique. TIVA can result in a faster turnaround time that may more than compensate for additional drug costs. Furthermore, there is no pollution of the operating theatre environment by vapours or gases.

Muscle relaxants

Muscle relaxants are not routinely used in day-case anaesthesia. However, a syringe of suxamethonium should be drawn up and available for all day-case anaesthetic sessions for emergency use, e.g. in laryngeal spasm.

Mivacurium chloride is a muscle relaxant particularly well-suited for day surgery. It is a non-depolarising muscle relaxant with a short duration of action. Its use does not cause muscle pains, and its duration of action is three times that of suxamethonium.

Adverse effects of anaesthetics

Post-operative nausea and vomiting (PONV) are common and distressing symptoms that assume greater importance in the day surgery setting. Sickness has economic implications, due to both the prophylactic use of anti-emetic drugs and an increased hospital admission rate. The causes of PONV are multifactorial, but it may be dramatically reduced by using appropriate anaesthetic techniques:

- TIVA with propofol and alfentanil;
- use of the Laryngeal Mask Airway;
- avoidance of muscle relaxants and their subsequent reversal;
- widespread use of local analgesia.

Simple means, such as limiting pharyngeal suction, moving patients slowly and keeping them warm may also reduce the problem. If patients are identified as being at risk of developing PONV on pre-operative assessment, the use of a prophylactic anti-emetic is indicated. Three anti-emetics routinely used are droperidol, metoclopramide and ondansetron.

Training

It is essential that nurses working in the recovery area have received sufficient training in the skills they will be required to practise. In day surgery, the recovery nurse may be required to work alone at times, thus the need for expertise is increased. A background in recovery nursing, anaesthetic nursing or intensive care nursing is vital for at least one member of the team. This guarantees training for further staff. Current resuscitation procedures and practice are mandatory. It is important to have a member of staff taking charge and leading the recovery area. This will ensure that practices will be standardised, audited and altered as necessary.

Recovery rooms save lives, enable staff to gain and maintain specialised skills, concentrate skilled staff in one area and prevent the duplication of equipment.

It is a common belief that patients are 'asleep' during an operation. They are not asleep, they have been put into a coma with drugs and it takes some hours for their bodies to recover. It is during this recovery period that the patient slowly becomes conscious and regains his protective reflexes. Before recovery rooms were routinely available, almost half the deaths in the immediate post-operative period were due to preventable causes, such as airway obstruction or aspiration of stomach contents.

Good recovery rooms improve patient safety, save money and allow the wards to work effectively.

Commentary

Some concluding comments by Judge Dohm in a Canadian malpractice case.

> The function of this room (the recovery room) is to provide highly specialised care and frequent and careful observation of the patients who are under the influence of anaesthesia. They remain in this room until they have regained consciousness and their bodies return to normal function. Respiratory arrest is not an uncommon occurrence in the recovery room and therefore the personnel in this room must be watchful and alert at all times in order to protect the patient in this labile and vulnerable stage. The nurses in this room are there for the purpose of promptly recognising any respiratory problem, cardiovascular problem or haemorrhaging. They are expected to take corrective action and/or to summon help promptly ... it is my opinion that the recovery room is the most important room in the hospital and the one in which the patient requires the greatest attention because it is fraught with the greatest potential danger to the patient. This known hazard carries with it, in my opinion, a higher degree of duty owed by the hospital to the patient ... close scrutiny and ever-present watchfulness is required in this room and the patient is entitled to expect the same.

It could not be said better.

Further reading

Hatfield A, Transon M (1996) The Complete Recovery Room Book. Oxford: Oxford Medical Publications.

Ogg TW, Wilson BJ (1995) Anaesthesia Rounds-Aspects of Day Surgery and Anaesthesia. Zeneca, England

Emergency situations and treatment

Airway obstruction

Causes

Face – closed/swollen lips, blocked nose, oedema
Mouth – teeth, foreign body, oedema
Pharynx – tonsils and adenoids, tongue, dentures, oedema, secretions, blood/vomit, laryngospasm
Larynx – trauma, injection, epiglottis, tumour, foreign body
Bronchi – secretions, clot, sputum, oedema
Bronchioles – irritable airways, chronic obstructive airways disease, allergic response

SIGNS

Total obstruction	Partial obstruction
No breath sounds	Noisy breathing
No movement of air or mask misting	Diminished air movement
Unco-ordinated paradoxical breathing pattern	Snoring,crowing wheezing, gurgling
Signs of hypoxia, cyanosis, falling SaO$_2$	Laboured breathing
Restlessness, confusion leading to loss of consciousness	
Cardiac dysrhythmias, cardiac bradycardia, arrest	

ACTION

Total obstruction	Partial obstruction
Chinlift, jaw thrust clean airway/ suction thrust/airway	thrust/airway
Jaw Suction	Jaw Suction
O$_2$ at 10–15 litres per minute	O$_2$ Chinlift, jaw thrust clean airway/ suction
Place patient in Left lateral position with head down	Place patient in Left lateral position with head down
Monitor vital signs	Monitor vital signs
Get help – emergency button	If condition deteriorates get help

If no improvement
Ventilate with ambu circuit
Emergency intubation trolley
with suxamethonium/atropine
Assist with emergency intubation

2. Partial to total airway occlusion

Laryngospasm in semi-conscious patient	**Laryngeal oedema**
CAUSES	
Use of endotracheal tube Stimulation of larynx on emergence from anaesthesia Blood/secretions on the larynx Clumsy extubation	Associated with operations on larynx
SIGNS	
Inspiratory stridor (crowing) See-saw breathing Laboured breathing Distressed patient Deterioration in colour	Distressed patient
ACTION	
Chin lift, jaw thrust Clear airway/suction O_2 via mask, 10–15 litres per minute or bag with 100% O_2 Suction via laryngoscope visualise cords to remove secretions Place patient in left lateral position Monitor vital signs	Sit patient up to reduce swelling Intravenous dexamethasone Helium/oxygen mixture Bag with re-breathing circuit Sedation

If larynx is clear but spasm persists

oxygenate with re-breathing bag	If condition deteriorates get help
If condition deteriorates prepare for emergency intubation	If intubation is impossible due to oedema, prepare for emergency cricothyroidotomy (mini tracheostomy)

3. Post-operative respiratory complications

Inadequate ventilation

CAUSES

Inadequate reversal from anaesthesia

Intravenous neostigmine to reverse muscle relaxants

Caused by opiates given pre- or peri-operatively; barbiturates, inhalation of anaesthesia; low respiratory drive

SIGNS

Rapid, shallow breathing
Minimal chest movement

'Floppy' muscle tone
Restlessness 'twitching'
Unco-ordinated limb movement
No control over respirations, movement

Test for hand grip, raising head from pillow, sticking out tongue. Patient will not have muscle tone to do these

Delayed return to consciousness
Respiratory rate less than 10 breaths per minute
Shallow breaths
Constricted pupils
Deterioration in colour

ACTION

Call for anaesthetist
Control airway
Administer oxygen
Monitor vital signs
Position:
lateral if semi-conscious;
prone/sitting up if conscious
Prepare and assist in administration of emergency drugs (see Chapter 4)

Control airway
Administer oxygen
Repeat as necessary
Monitor vital signs
Review analgesia
Prepare and assist in administration of emergency drugs (see Chapter 4)

Aspiration of gastric contents

During recovery from anaesthesia the laryngeal (epiglottal) reflex may be depressed. If vomiting/regurgitation occurs, gastric contents may be aspirated into lungs.

Avoid by ensuring all un/semi conscious patients lie on side in order that gastric contents drain out.

IF VOMITING OCCURS

Turn patient on side/head down for drainage
Apply suction to pharynx/use laryngoscope and magill forceps to remove solids
Administer oxygen at 10–15 litres via a face mask

IF ASPIRATION OCCURS FOLLOWING VOMITING

Patients will:
1. be intubated for intermittent positive pressure ventilation and suction of trachea
2. be administered antibiotics
3. have a chest X-ray
4. be monitored for vital signs
5. be transferred to ITU
6. have physiotherapy

Bronchospasm

Caused by irritation of larynx during emergence from anaesthesia from secretions, endotracheal tube, suction catheter. Smokers and asthmatics are at risk.

SIGNS

Dyspnoea
Wheezing
See-saw respirations
Deterioration in patient's colour-cyanosis

ACTION

Administer oxygen
Call for anaesthetist
Prepare bronchodilators
Sit patient up if possible

Chapter 6
Care of the patient in the day surgical unit

Basia Howard-Harwood

Introduction

The recent evolution and expansion of the day surgical service has direct implications on patients, health care professionals and the National Health Service as a whole. With the emphasis on self-care, day surgery challenges many traditional roles and perceptions of health care, and both service users and service providers need to adapt to face these challenges head on.

It is, therefore, not surprising that day surgery has direct implications on the surgical nurse, whose role lies at the forefront of service provision (Hodge, 1993). Day surgery nurses have an important role to play in this specialty, and are vital members of the multidisciplinary health care team, which encompasses staff from both the community and hospital environments. In no other specialty will the nurse be given such a good opportunity to develop skills and gain from the vast experiences offered by both the ward and theatre environments. Day surgery offers the surgical nurse a unique opportunity to provide comprehensive patient care, and to develop the nurse's role to meet the challenges of this specialty.

It is the evolution of modern analgesic and anaesthetic agents, which allow for patients' early mobilisation post-operatively (NHSME, 1991), and the development of minimally invasive surgical techniques and modern technology, that have made it possible for senior surgeons and anaesthetists to offer day surgery to their patients. This makes day surgery an 'economical, efficient and effective use of resources' (Markanday & Platzer, 1994, p. 38).

Day surgery has great potential for development within the current marketplace. With the emphasis on maintaining high standards of care, cost-effectiveness and competitiveness (Audit Commission, 1991a), day surgery is compatible with today's health service (Avis, 1992). Day surgery can increase the overall throughput of patients (Audit Commission, 1991b) and reduces hospital waiting lists by up to one third (Audit Commission, 1991a). Furthermore, day surgery is thought to be a resource capable of cutting costs in the NHS by up to 65 per cent (NHSME, 1991), and meeting standards outlined in the *Patients' Charter* (NHSME, 1993). Targets forecast that up to 50 per cent of all patients undergoing elective surgery could be considered appropriate candidates for day surgical admission for 1995–96 (NHS Executive, 1994).

Day surgery is not a passing phase. It is a new and exciting specialty that is growing steadily worldwide. It has opened up opportunities for nurses at all levels, from the Common Foundation Programme student nurse on a dip-in placement, to the qualified and more experienced staff nurse. The opportunity to work on the ward base and in the theatre setting, enables nurses to develop a range of specialised skills offered only by this field of nursing.

Although there is still scope for improvement, day surgery is a valid option open to patients faced with undergoing a range of elective surgical procedures. Furthermore, it is the day surgical nurse who is in the prime position to plan and provide the care that the patient requires. It is this specialised care that is explored in detail in this chapter.

Total care of the day surgery patient

The day surgery nurse holds a prime position in organising and providing the care for day surgery patients. The nurse prepares the patient both physically and psychologically for surgery, and for the subsequent discharge home. Although the multidisciplinary team work together to ensure the patient's smooth passage through the unit, it is the nurse who has the most contact and influence over the patient.

Because a day surgery patient's care is condensed into half a day, unique skills are required from nurses working in this specialty (NHSME, 1991). A combination of training, staff development and experience are required to ensure that the nurse will have the necessary knowledge and skills to fulfil this role, and as a result, be able to 'safeguard and promote the best interests of individual patients and clients' (UKCC, 1992b, para 6.1).

The day surgery nurse

Many patients coming to the unit are new to the hospital environment and find the prospect of day surgery rather daunting. It is the nurse who can counsel patients and prepare them for the experiences that lie ahead. In a very short space of time, the nurse must establish and develop a good rapport with their patients. A friendly manner and good communication skills are an essential combination for this to be achieved. Where a good nurse–patient relationship has been established, a patient is more likely to ask questions about aspects of care he or she does not understand (Kempe, 1987), and this can only benefit the patient. The information received can make the surgery less stressful for the patient, and should reduce the level of anxiety felt about admission (Haines, 1992). The nurse also needs to use appropriate communication skills to communicate effectively within the multidisciplinary team and act as an advocate for the patient, and, in turn, to promote the patient's best interests.

As well as having good communication skills, nurses need to be able to support the patient's psychological needs and provide emotional support, which can help to prepare a patient for early discharge.

As health care practitioners, nurses are accountable for all aspects of care given to patients, and the care must be based on an accurate assessment of needs. The assessment needs to be rational, systematic and goal-directed, and could be made by using the framework of a nursing care plan. Any written plan must demonstrate awareness of the problems an individual patient may encounter. Furthermore, the nursing care plan will allow the nurse to plan, implement and, finally, evaluate the level of patient care delivered. This area is explored fully later in the chapter.

The role of teacher and educator is a crucial component of the day surgical nurse's role. By using every given opportunity to inform and educate patients about what to expect both at the unit, and on discharge, the nurse can increase a patient's ability to provide self-care post-operatively.

More and more patients are being encouraged to contribute towards meeting their own health care needs, and education encourages the day surgical patient to take a more active role in this care. Where a partnership between the patient and nurse emerges, the nurse can use her or his knowledge and skills to increase a patient's level of understanding, which in turn will promote the patient's recovery to health (Henderson, 1988).

Increasing a patient's level of knowledge and understanding, increases compliance with post-operative instructions and reduces the likelihood of post-operative complications (Haines, 1992). This is a desired outcome; non-compliance can cause post-operative complications to arise in the home following discharge, and complications are likely to reduce a patient's satisfaction with the service and his or her ability to cope with self-care in the home. Furthermore, patient education can reduce the physical and psychological impact of surgery at both the pre- and post-operative stages (Kempe, 1987), and as professional practitioners, nurses have a duty of care to educate patients so that they are able to look after themselves following discharge. Because of the inherent time restrictions of day surgery, there is much less time available in which to pass on information to the patient, and the nurse, who sees the patient from pre-assessment to discharge, needs to make good use of the limited time available.

No two patients have the same level of prior knowledge or capacity for learning, and learning will only occur if the teaching is tailored to the individual's needs (Farrelly & Lakeman, 1993). For teaching to be a success, the nurse needs first to assess each patient's knowledge and motivation to learn. The nurse needs to make good use of her or his teaching strategies, as learning will not occur unless the patient is motivated and recognises the need for new information.

Clearly educating patients is not an easy task. It is a skill that 'requires an understanding of human behaviour and an appreciation that there is more to learning than just receiving information' (Farrelly & Lakeman, 1993, p. 19). This topic is explored further later in the chapter.

From all this, it is quite clear that the day surgery nurse has an important and demanding role to perform as an educator, supporter, counsellor, carer, communicator, assessor and advocate. The nurse's role is truly multidisciplinary, and she or he must deliver care and use her or his skills in all of the day surgery's settings.

In the pre-assessment clinic the nurse undertakes the patient's pre-operative screening, and checks each individual's suitability for early discharge. On the ward prior to surgery, the nurse welcomes the patient to the unit and prepares him or her for the surgery ahead. In theatre, the nurse helps the anaesthetist, assists the surgeon, circulates and cares for the patient during the recovery period. On the ward post-operatively, the nurse provides care for the patient and ensures safe discharge criteria are met before the patient is allowed to leave the unit. Throughout the unit, nurses provide their patients with a high level of comprehensive care, which clearly encompasses the total care of the day surgery patient.

Continuity of care

Clearly no one nurse can see a patient through all these areas in a single day. It is up to the nursing team to provide continuity of care throughout the ward, theatre and recovery areas. Nurses should have the necessary skills to rotate internally through these areas of clinical practice, as internal rotation and total patient care are thought to generate good team spirit, improve a nurse's job satisfaction, and be an efficient and economical use of staff (Penn, 1993).

In the author's unit, experience and skill-development in ward and theatre practice are crucial and staff development a priority. Ideally, nurses should follow a comprehensive orientation package in both ward and theatre environments, which should give them the competence and skills needed to rotate successfully at intervals between the different day surgery areas. A note of concern was, however, recently expressed by Sutherland (1994, p. 12), who urged caution of any nurse who would claim 'mastery' over all the separate specialties of day surgery. By promoting a 'supernurse' role, Sutherland felt nurses would run the risk of delivering substandard care to their patients and be in danger of threatening their profession by claiming expertise in several areas of practice despite relatively limited experience.

In the author's experience, nurses who have had experience in all areas of day surgery provide for a flexible and co-operative workforce. Within the confines of the day surgical unit (DSU), nurses are safe and competent practitioners able to meet patients' needs from the ward through to theatre, provided they have received appropriate training and education. Caution should be exercised such that a patient's care and best interests are always a priority, and no nurse should undertake a role which she or he is not qualified to fulfil. The nurse's role must always serve the best interests of the patient and any 'enlargement or adjustment of the scope of personal professional practice must be achieved without compromising or fragmenting existing aspects of professional practice and care, and that the requirements of the Council's Code of Professional Conduct are satisfied throughout the whole area of practice' (UKCC, 1992a, para 9.4).

Check-list or care plan?

A care plan allows the nurse to use the nursing process to assess the patient's needs and plan appropriate care. By using the framework of a care plan for guidance, a nurse can assess, plan, implement and evaluate each patient's individualised care. The care plan acts as a record of a patient's care and can be used as a memory aid to prevent omissions. Although similarities between the care plans of patients undergoing the same procedure are unavoidable, the nurse can indi-vidualise the plan to address the particular needs of each patient.

The day surgery care plan allows the nurse responsible for providing a patient's care to record all interventions taken, as the record follows the patient from pre-assessment through to discharge home. Be it on the ward, in theatre or recovery, the care plan acts as means for members of the nursing team to communicate with each other. Furthermore, when a nurse signs for care given in any area, she or he accepts responsibility for action taken.

In the author's unit the care plan states the unit's nursing goal. This is that every patient assessed will have their individual self-care needs and deficits identified, and that each patient will be discharged home having recovered sufficiently from surgery and having been empowered to meet his or her own self-care needs.

The favoured nursing framework for day surgery from which the care plan is written is the self-care model coined by Orem (1991). In this model, the goal is to provide self-care as quickly as possible. To achieve this, any deficits in self-care that result from the surgery or the anaesthetic must be addressed, so that the patient can be safely discharged home able to meet his or her own self-care needs. The nurse's role is to help the patient by acting as an educator, supporter and representative, and by establishing a developmental environ-ment (Vasquez, 1992).

The model is based on four components – person, health, envi-ronment and nursing. Care provision is only a transient stage, as the goal of guiding a person to self-care dominates. Orem (1991) describes three types of self-care requisites – universal, developmental and health deviation. These are considered fundamental to human existence. A nurse can act for a patient at different stages of his or her stay on the day surgery unit, and the nurse's actions in dealing with the patient's self-care deficits will vary accordingly, from wholly compensatory to partly compensatory to educative-developmental. The nurse prepares the patient and his or her family to assume responsibility for self-care on discharge from the unit (Vasquez, 1992). On a patient's care record the nurse should record the patient's personal details and a telephone number for the next of kin.

At pre-assessment, a nurse will assess the patient's universal self-care needs in the categories of air, water/food, elimination, prevention of hazards, promotion of normality, mobility and social interaction. This assessment will act as the basis for the patient's care. On admission to the unit on the day of surgery, the nurse will check for any deviation from the initial assessment and prepare the patient for theatre. The nurse completes a pre-operative check-list to ensure that all appropriate actions have been taken.

The patient is than taken to theatre, where nurses document their wholly compensatory actions. In recovery, the patient moves through to a partly compensatory stage, which continues in varying degrees until the patient returns to the ward. On the ward, the nurse assesses the patient's potential and actual health deviation self-care needs and the nursing actions required. This may be that the patient must tolerate diet and fluid by discharge, or for the nurse to give full advice on analgesia to the patient and his or her escort. A final area of the care plan is completed on discharge from the unit when the patient's care is evaluated by the discharge nurse. The ultimate aim is for the patient to have recovered sufficiently from surgery to meet his or her own self-care needs on discharge.

Managing potential anxiety

Patient anxiety and its management is often considered to be a crucial part of the day surgical nurse's role, and as such is fully discussed later in the chapter. However, some doubts were recently raised as to whether or not reducing anxiety through information-giving, was always beneficial to the patient.

One opinion, is that patients can only benefit from information – people who have no interest in the information given will ignore it and, as such, cannot be harmed by it (Bysshe, 1988). In contrast, Salmon (1993) suggested that it was wrong to assume that reducing a patient's anxiety would automatically aid recovery, as moderate levels of anxiety could help prepare patients for surgery and, in turn, reduce stress.

In the author's experience, most patients appear to benefit from health education and anxiety management. However, in view of these findings, it may be appropriate that, in some cases, nurses use their discretion for 'teaching only that which is essential ... for those with a low preference for information in order to avoid creating more stress in an already stressful situation' (Caldwell, 1991, p. 181).

New role for patient and staff

Day surgery relies on new roles being undertaken by both nurses and patients. Day surgery nurses need to allow their patients more autonomy and encourage greater responsibility for patient-led post-operative care. To achieve this, the nurse must have an understanding of her or his facilitative and empowering role, and demonstrate an awareness of the challenges facing the patient. Nurses can learn this new philosophy by combining day surgical experience with training and education, and by undertaking specialist day surgery ENB courses. It is then up to the nurse to move the patient from the traditionally dependent role, through a partnership in care, towards self-care on discharge.

Successful care in the day surgery unit relies on a shift in responsibility from nurses to patients and their families. Patients are expected to participate in their care and to have an understanding of the choices available to them. Traditionally, patients were conditioned into a passive role by their nurse, who would assume a dominant role in the nurse–patient relationship. However, patients are now expected to work in partnership with their nurse and to take some responsibility for their own care.

Some patients may find their role in the relationship uncomfortable, preferring to remain passive and to hold no responsibility in making any decisions (Avis, 1992). It must be remembered that 'although the idea of patient participation and partnership remains desirable in terms of promoting autonomy, patients appear not to expect such a role in their relationship with health professionals' (Avis, 1992, p. 10).

Clearly, patients and nurses still need to undergo a culture change before fully accepting day surgery and the changed dynamics within the nurse–patient relationship.

In addition to the implications for the day surgical nurse and her or his role, it is important to consider the implications that day surgery may have for the traditional surgical nurse's role. As a result of all minor in-patient cases being treated in a day surgery setting, nurses working on traditional wards will inadvertently have a heavier workload of major cases (Bridger & Rees,1995). This, in turn, may have implications for their functioning as a team and may result in a need to renegotiate staffing level and existing skill mix.

Some patients undergoing day surgery, have unrealistic expectations and beliefs about the service offered. Because of the short length of stay in hospital, many patients think that the severity of surgery has been reduced and that a full recovery to health will occur prior to discharge (Dutton, 1994). In this instance, it is the nurse's responsibility to inform the patient of the implications of day surgery and the subsequent time period required for post-operative recovery.

Local anaesthetic patients

Nursing care for patients undergoing a local anaesthetic is condensed into the short length of time the patient is in the unit, which, on average, is between two and four hours. Because patients are not routinely pre-assessed prior to admission the nurse must be sure to use all the time available appropriately to facilitate the patient's safe passage through the unit, to discharge home.

The nursing care given to local anaesthetic patients is similar to, though not as detailed as, that given to general anaesthetic cases. Furthermore, specialist skills are required of the nurse to help the patient cope with his or her admission. The same documentation as that for general anaesthetic cases is used, though in less detail, enabling the nurse to assess the patient's psychological, physical and social circumstances. On admission, patients are told what they can expect to happen during their time on the unit and what precautions they should follow on discharge home.

Patients need to be reassured early on that the only discomfort they will experience while in theatre will be the local anaesthetic being administered into the operation site, and that surgery will not begin unless sensation is no longer experienced. Patients should also be reassured that they will not see the surgery being performed and that a theatre nurse will sit and talk with them while surgery is in progress. Furthermore, patients need to be educated that despite being carried out under a local anaesthetic, the severity of surgery should not be dismissed. One patient on the author's unit having an inguinal hernia repair, had planned a day's golf one day after surgery, and was very disappointed when the nurse informed him that he was restricted from mobilising in the same way as if he had undergone a general anaesthetic.

On discharge, patients should receive full discharge information from their nurse and advice about pain management. Because most patients leave the unit pain-free due to the continuing effects of local anaesthetic, the nurse needs to be firm in giving advice about analgesia. In general, patients should be advised to use regular analgesia for up to 48 hours post-operatively, regardless of whether they feel they need to or not.

Special needs of elderly patients

For many elderly patients day surgery is a foreign concept, but if they are given adequate reassurance and support, many prefer the option of day surgery. They experience fewer changes to their daily routines and are less likely to be confused because they do not need to stay overnight in an unfamiliar hospital ward (Davies & Ogg, 1993). However, elderly patients are often excluded from the DSU because they do not meet all the set physical, psychological or social criteria for general or local anaesthetic admission. Elderly patients are more likely to have a disabled or incapacitated carer who is unable to provide transport or adequate support after discharge. Family and friends may not always be able to intervene due to their own commitments. Furthermore, travelling to the hospital for pre-assessment and for surgery may incur considerable expense for patients in this age-group, as a volunteer hospital driver cannot always be arranged. As a result, such simple criteria as post-operative care or transport home from the hospital can be obstacles to surgery being performed, and even simple limb surgery can compromise the patient's safety and independence once home (Farquharson, 1993).

In certain circumstances it may be possible to overcome these obstacles. Some patients with impaired vision may benefit from being given advice sheets with larger print, to increase ease of reading. Short-term home care and community nursing support can be arranged through the patient's general practitioner (GP), to give the patient additional support. These measures, when combined with good psychological preparation, appropriate information and community support, can enable some elderly people to be safely admitted and discharged from the DSU.

Patient satisfaction

In line with the increased awareness of accountability within the NHS, there has been an increase in the level of review of patient satisfaction (Bowling, 1993). Satisfaction can influence a day surgery patient's adherence to treatment and compliance with post-operative regimens (Bowling, 1993).The Audit Commission (1991a) identified a need for individual DSUs to monitor patients' attitudes and review satisfaction with services provided.

In a recent report, 80 per cent of people questioned expressed a preference to be treated within day-care criteria (Audit Commission, 1991b). Patient satisfaction is vital in the free NHS market and to the continuing success of day surgery. Improvements to the service should reflect not only staff opinions, but also patients' ideas and suggestions, and patient satisfaction should remain a priority and top any agenda.

Protocols and policy for discharge

Discharge planning and patient selection criteria are just two of the areas where individual day surgery units benefit from setting out their aims for practice within documented operational policies. Once set out, these guidelines should be followed by the staff working in the unit (Medical Defence Union, 1992), thus ensuring that patients benefit from a given standard of care. The report by the Day Surgery Task Force (NHSME, 1993) sets out clear guidelines on what the contents of an operational policy should be. Such a policy should advise on good working practice and reflect the individual unit's overall philosophy for care.

At the time of a patient's discharge from the unit, it is crucial that meticulous attention to detail be followed. It is only if appropriate and effective working practice has been followed and policies have been strictly adhered to, that the patient can be safely discharged home after day surgery. A patient who has not been properly prepared for discharge home by the nurse is unlikely to be safe post-operatively and may be unable to cope with self-care in the home environment. Then, as a direct consequence of discharge protocols not being strictly adhered to, the nurse will have failed in her or his responsibility of ensuring a patient's safety on discharge, and the overall success of the day surgical service may become compromised.

Clearly, good discharge planning is crucial to day surgery and should begin early, at the patient's pre-assessment visit. During a pre-assessment visit, the nurse assesses the patient's suitability for under-going a surgical procedure within day-care criteria. In doing this, the nurse is also assessing whether or not the patient is likely to be able to be safely discharged home within one working day. Carrington (1993, p. 12) saw careful patient selection as 'an essential prerequisite for safe day surgery', making this aspect of the service a crucial and important part of the day surgical process.

It is during the pre-assessment visit that the nurse is able to make an assessment of the patient's medical, psychological and social status (Reynolds & Morgan, 1991). Medically, a patient must be physically fit to undergo a general anaesthetic and subsequently fit for discharge home within a couple of hours of returning to the ward after surgery. Psychologically, a patient's fears and anxieties need to be identified at pre-assessment so that the nurse can help the patient with early discharge. Furthermore, patient's individual concerns will need to be addressed and the preparatory process behind early discharge implemented. Finally, the nurse needs to assess the patient's social circumstances. The patient must have adequate social support available post-operatively to ensure that his or her safety following discharge is not compromised in the event of anaes-thetic or surgical complications.

Discharge criteria

Many units' patient discharge criteria are based on guidelines proposed by the Royal College of Surgeons Report of the Working Party on Guidelines for Day Surgery (1992). The Report advocates the use of written advice sheets to reinforce verbal information given to patients, and suggests that all patients benefit from receiving advice specifically related to the surgery they have undergone. An example of this may be to advise a patient who has undergone a termination of pregnancy to avoid sexual intercourse for two weeks to reduce the risk of infection. All patients who have undergone a general anaesthetic are advised against operating machinery (which includes driving and using kitchen appliances), signing legally binding documents and making important decisions for 48 hours following surgery.

On discharge, patients leaving the unit should be told when and with whom follow-up appointments have been arranged. Depending on the nature and extent of surgery, some patients will need no other follow-up than to attend their GP's surgery for the removal of sutures or to have their wound checked; others will need to attend further consultations with their surgeon in the hospital out-patients department. Patients also need to be aware of whom to contact in case post-operative complications are experienced once home. They may be advised to seek advice or assistance from the community nursing service, their GP, or simply to return to the hospital and see the on-call surgeon from the appropriate surgical team.

Despite every effort to screen patients' suitability for early discharge at pre-assessment, in some circumstances patients may be unfit to go home following surgery. If this should happen, whether for anaesthetic or surgical reasons, provision must be made for overnight admission. Patients who are not fit for discharge should not be forced home, but every effort should be made to transfer them into an overnight bed, preferably on a ward dealing with their specialty.

Finally, before leaving the unit, the Royal College of Surgeons Report (1992) also suggests that patients' suitability for discharge should be assessed by a medical officer. Clearly, this may not always be possible in practice. The Report acknowledges this, and accepts that this responsibility could be delegated to the senior nursing sister in the unit. At this stage the patient's wound must be checked to ensure that the dressing is clean and intact, and an assessment must be made of the patient's general condition. As with all other stages of a day surgery patient's stay on the unit, this assessment needs to be clearly documented and recorded in the patient's records.

In the author's experience, these guidelines form only a basic framework for a day surgery unit's discharge policy, and more detailed criteria are often added by individual units to improve their patients' experiences, safeguard their wellbeing and ensure a safe passage through the day surgery unit. These criteria need to be set and agreed by the unit's multidisciplinary health care team. In the author's unit, strict acceptance criteria have been devised such that the service is offered only to those patients who are felt to be able to cope with early discharge.

Any surgery lasting longer than one hour is not normally performed as a day case. Similarly, patients suffering from a chronic illness are not accepted for day surgery. Any underlying medical condition must be well controlled and advice sought from the consultant anaesthetist before accepting the patient for day surgery (for further details of this see Chapter 3).

Relationship between pre-assessment and safe discharge

Chapter 2 discussed the issue of pre-assessment and briefly explored discharge planning. This section aims to identify the vital role pre-assessment plays in the safe discharge of the day surgical patient.

At pre-assessment, patients are questioned about their home circumstances to ensure that they will have adequate post-operative support after discharge. A responsible adult must escort the patient home in a private car or taxi, and stay and care for the patient for 24 hours post-operatively. This is done to ensure that someone is on hand to assist or initiate a call for help if surgical or anaesthetic complications were to arise in the immediate post-operative period. In the author's unit a patient who has undergone a hernia repair is, for the first 48 hours, allowed out of bed only to use the toilet. Therefore, a carer must be on hand to provide comprehensive care in the patient's immediate post-operative period and to support the patient as required during convalescence, which may take up to 12 weeks.

The patient's journey home should take no longer than one hour. Furthermore, patients should have access to an inside toilet, and anyone who has had lower limb surgery should not have to climb stairs to get home. In some cases, patients may be asked to arrange to stay with friends post-operatively to overcome any potential hazards identified. For others, it may be appropriate to arrange for a physiotherapist to teach the patient to use crutches and climb stairs post-operatively.

Information-giving is initiated at pre-assessment and patients should be told what to expect on the day of surgery and how to manage once home. Information sheets are useful to reinforce all that is said about post-operative management, the unit and its routines, and pre-operative regimens. For surgery such as the stripping of varicose veins or hernia repair, where nursing care may be transferred to the community nursing service, an initial referral can be made to the community nurse through the community liaison staff. Naturally, the patient should be informed of this referral at pre-assessment.

Where pre-assessment is routinely performed for all patients, the nurse's task at discharge is considerably easier. The patient has already received discharge information and the necessary plans for discharge are in place. An informed patient is happier and calmer, and at no other time is this more evident than at discharge.

Guidelines in assessment for discharge

In the author's unit, policies additional to those set by the Royal College of Surgeons (1992) are used to guide the nurse at the actual time of a patient's discharge. These policies further increase the desired outcome of a patient's successful early discharge.

All patients will have tolerated a drink and a snack on the unit prior to discharge, and any nausea or vomiting will be controlled. Patients are advised that any post-operative nausea and vomiting could continue for up to 48 hours, but the incidence of this has been greatly reduced by the use of new, lighter anaesthetic agents. Pain will be within tolerable limits from oral analgesia and the patient will be physically capable of walking out of the unit and will be observed by the nurse walking in a straight line. Any post-operative bleeding must be well controlled and patients are advised against driving for 48 hours. Patients should be advised that this is an important consideration, because an accident that occurs during this post-operative period could leave them uninsured in the event of an insurance claim.

All discharge information given at pre-assessment is reinforced with both the patient and escort present. The only exception to this may arise in the case of a patient who has undergone a termination of pregnancy, where the escort may be unaware of the surgery performed. In this case, the nurse may find it more appropriate to give any information to the patient alone. When the nurse discharges the patient the information she is giving is reinforcement and revision and is, therefore, more likely to be retained and remembered.

All patients leaving the unit should be given a letter for their GP. The patient should be advised to keep the letter at home overnight in case any problems occur in the immediate post-operative period. Should none arise, this letter can then be taken to the surgery.

Local anaesthetic discharge criteria

Many units do not set an upper age limit for patients, although those over the age of 75 are often not medically fit enough to undergo a day-case general anaesthetic. In some such cases, if the social and psychological criteria have been met, and if the procedure allows, patients can have the surgery performed under a local anaesthetic.

Unlike general anaesthetic cases, most patients attending the unit to have surgery under a local anaesthetic are not pre-assessed. In some DSUs patients over 70 are pre-assessed in their homes by a member of the community nursing team. However, most patients are just sent written advice through the post, giving information about the unit, the day surgery routine and post-operative regimens advocated, and this is usually an adequate measure. However, where a breakdown in communication between the hospital and community teams has occurred, or in the event of an unsuitable patient being referred and placed on a theatre list, problems that pre-assessment would have identified may arise.

Some patients face the disappointment of being refused surgery on the day and then having to wait their turn on an in-patient waiting list. Alternatively, if surgery is performed, the patient may need to be admitted onto a ward overnight. Inevitably, there will be some patients attending the unit to have an operation under local anaesthetic who would benefit from pre-assessment at the unit. This is currently an area of great debate, and it is explored further in Chapter 2.

Discharge policies for patients undergoing local and general anaesthetics differ. Most local anaesthetic cases are able to leave the unit within one hour of returning to the ward after the procedure has been completed. As with general anaesthetic cases, the wound is checked, post-operative information is reinforced and patients are given the opportunity to ask questions. Patients are advised against driving themselves home from the unit, but they are not restricted from operating machinery in the home for 48 hours because they will not experience anaesthetic side effects and, therefore, safety will not be compromised. Similarly, although an escort home is required, the patient does not need 24-hour supervision as in the case of a general anaesthetic.

Most patients who have undergone a local anaesthetic will not experience any pain on discharge from the unit. This is because the effects of the local anaesthetic will block the patient's perception of pain. However, patients should be warned of this, and advised that unless analgesics are used, pain may become intolerable when the local anaesthetic wears off.

Local anaesthetics are not just an option open to those who are medically unsuitable for a general anaesthetic. It is a cost-effective method for many surgical procedures, and its use, without doubt, will become more widespread in future years.

Support for the patient after discharge

Over the past 10 years, much has been written about the benefits experienced by day surgery patients as a result of their early discharge from the unit. Early discharge has been credited with reducing the incidence of hospital-acquired wound infections (NHSME, 1991) and reducing the risk of post-operative thrombolytic complications (RCS, 1985). Furthermore, day surgery avoids prolonged family separation, which is thought to contribute towards a patient's faster post-operative recovery to health (NHSME, 1993). It is also important to remember that most patients express a preference for day surgery as opposed to a conventional in-patient admission because they would rather recover at home than on a hospital ward (Markanday & Platzer, 1994).

However, when discussing the benefits of early discharge, it is equally important to consider both the disadvantages and the advantages facing the patient. A study by Senapati and Young (1989) highlighted three areas that could put day surgical patients at a disadvantage to their in-patient counterparts. These were the incidence and management of post-operative complications, higher patient anxiety and poor pain management. Clearly, all three areas could hinder the success of a patient's early discharge from the unit, and it is important that these issues are addressed by the day surgical staff so as to improve patients' experiences and to ensure that the success of early discharge is not compromised.

Overcoming the disadvantages

Managing post-operative bleeding or any other post-operative complication is, on the whole, likely to be better managed in hospital rather than in the community. However, the incidence of such complications can be reduced by employing staff with experience and expertise in this field. Patients who have benefited from specialist medical and nursing care are thought to be less likely to develop these complications post-operatively (Hodge, 1994). However, patients need to be told whom they can contact for help if any problems do arise. This may be the community nursing service, their GP, or they may simply be told to return to the hospital and seek advice from the surgical team.

A common obstacle facing the day surgical patient after discharge is post-operative pain management. Although patients are warned to expect post-operative pain at pre-assessment, many underestimate the level of pain they will experience. Some patients believe that because they are discharged on the day of surgery the operation is less serious than a conventional in-patient admission, and consequently, that any pain experienced will be negligible. These patients then find that they are unprepared for managing their pain once home.

Post-operative pain can cause many unwanted physical and psychological side effects. Post-operative pain is associated with raised blood pressure and pulse, causing muscle tension, irritability and withdrawal. Furthermore, nausea and vomiting can interfere with a patient's food and fluid intake, which will lead to increased tiredness and reluctance to mobilise (Dale, 1993). Pain can also interfere with memory, thus preventing the patient from remembering post-operative information (Haines & Viellion, 1990).

At pre-assessment, nurses forewarn their patients of post-operative pain and discuss its management. Patients are advised to have oral analgesics available at home, as the unit gives only a limited number of days' supply of painkillers on discharge. In the immediate post-operative period nurses need constantly to re-assess their patients' pain. The effectiveness of any analgesics dispensed must be documented, and a pain scale can be used to gauge the level of a patient's pain (Dale, 1993). Seers (1987) suggested that nurses, on occasion, underestimate a patient's pain, and so it is important that nurses remain objective when making this assessment.

Many patients leave hospital pain-free because of local anaesthetic blocks. On discharge, all patients are advised to take analgesics regularly for between 24 and 48 hours post-operatively, and not to wait for pain levels to escalate. Patients can also help to control their pain by resting, elevating any affected limb and following specific advice given by the nursing staff on discharge. This can help to improve pain control and keep pain at a tolerable level.

The final area of concern facing the day surgical patient is anxiety management. During admission to the DSU patients may suffer from an increase in anxiety. A patient whose fears and worries have not been allayed while at the unit, is likely to remain anxious and lack confidence on discharge home. However, by providing the patient with health education and information, the nurse can allay the patient's fears and reduce anxiety for discharge home.

Day surgery nurses help prepare their patients to meet their self-care needs through an ongoing education programme. By giving a combination of written and verbal information, the nurse empowers the patient and his or her carer and reduces their anxiety about discharge (Mitchell, 1994). The verbal information given to the patient on discharge is a reinforcement of what was said at pre-assessment, so that the patient is reminded of the restrictions facing him or her on return home. The patient is also made aware of potential complications that may arise, and is advised on appropriate action to take should assistance be required.

Effective patient education can improve the overall quality of a patient's care and improve compliance with post-operative regimens (Haines, 1992). When verbal and written information are used together, one reinforces the other and may increase a patient's retention of information. The subject matter must be relevant to the patient as 'what patients really want to know can all too easily be overlooked by professionals ... if you give patients the information they want, everybody wins' (Rickford & Lyall, 1995, p. 5). Furthermore, written information may remind a patient of verbal advice given, which may otherwise have been forgotten because of pain or anxiety (Dobree, 1989).

To improve a patient's understanding and to be a good educational tool, information sheets needs to be written in a simple format, using only simple terms (Farrelly & Lakeman, 1994). Medical jargon should be avoided, but caution must be exercised not to oversimplify language and risk putting across a patronising message (Dobree, 1989). Despite the obvious advantages, written information is often not read by patients. Thus, staff must encourage patients to read the information given and to follow the advice suggested.

Community nursing service

Any nursing care required by the patient following discharge tends to be taken over by the community nursing service. In some cases, patients are automatically referred by the day surgical unit to the community nurse, while in others, the GP may refer a patient only if a problem arises. In some hospitals, community liaison staff visit the day surgical unit to collect any patient referrals for the community nurses. Patients are referred to the community nurse working for their primary health care team, and either visits or telephone calls are made to check on a patient's progress.

At pre-assessment, nurses make an initial referral to the community nursing team, so as to inform the community staff of a patient's proposed surgery. This referral is then confirmed on the day of the patient's admission, so that the community nurse can plan her or his workload accordingly. Patients who are referred to the community nursing service are warned that they will receive a home visit or a telephone call from the nurse on the day following surgery. If, however, the patient requires nursing assistance or advice overnight, one option is to use a 'twilight' nursing service. The patient is given a contact telephone number on discharge from the unit so that he or she can benefit from community nursing support 24 hours a day.

There is a need for co-operation and for open communication channels to exist between the hospital and community teams. One way of achieving this is through a liaison group, with multidisciplinary representation from both areas of clinical practice. Here, protocols and discharge policies can be negotiated and agreed, and both teams can work to meet the same goal.

With the increase in numbers and the complexity of day case surgery, community staff have experienced an increase in their workload. It can be argued that day surgery may have transferred costs and responsibility away from the hospital and onto the community. This is a concern voiced by some GPs, and clearly, if the patient is to continue to receive the same level of community support, there may be a need for a review of the level of resources made available to the community staff (Bailey, 1993).

Currently, the community liaison nurse is responsible for co-ordinating care between the day surgical unit and the community. However, problems can arise if there is a breakdown in communication and community nurses are given incorrect patient details or late notification of any changes (Ruckley et al., 1980). This may result in patient support systems failing to provide the desired level of patient care. Furthermore, in some locations community nurse support following day surgery is limited and this may prevent some patients from undergoing day surgery. This could be avoided if day-based surgery nurses extended their care into the community. Jackson et al. (1993, p. 5) suggested that because of the increase in numbers of patients being treated as day cases 'there should be a change in who is responsible for their post-operative management'.

At the moment no provision is made for day surgery during a community nurse's training, therefore, it can be argued that the community nurse may not fully understand this specialty. The author believes that it is a valid option to consider extending the day surgical nurse's role into the community. By combining day surgical experience with community training a new role could be created so that the patient could benefit from nursing support directly from the day surgical unit.

Support after discharge

The NHS Management Executive (1993) set guidelines outlining a day surgical nurse's responsibility to patients. The guidelines made no reference to a nurse having any responsibility to patients following their discharge home from the unit. Ralphs (1994) claimed that day surgical nurses were responsible for their patients' care from assessment through to discharge home, at which point any further nursing support became the sole responsibility of the community nurse. However, a day surgery-led post-discharge follow-up is now standard practice and widely accepted in the USA (Burden, 1992), where day surgery facilitates the majority of all elective surgical procedures performed.

Young (1990, p. 273) saw a post-operative follow-up telephone call to be an 'essential part' of the day surgical nurse's responsibility. From this, a nurse could make an evaluation of the patient's physical and psychological health, 'thus completing the nursing process' (Burden, 1992, p. 259) and ensuring that all responsibility to the patient had been met. The nurse is considered to be the most appropriate member of the day surgical team to carry out this intervention because of her or his knowledge of the surgical procedures performed. Furthermore, she or he is capable of using professional judgements when evaluating health information given by the patient during the telephone call (Burden, 1992).

Nurses are capable of providing the patient with additional information if further problems are identified (Young, 1990), and are able to pass on unresolved queries to the appropriate member of the multidisciplinary health care team (Burden, 1992). By providing this support following a patient's discharge home, the nurse improves the patient's continuity of care and can further decrease a patient's anxiety (Kempe & Gelazis, 1985).

Despite a concerted effort by nurses to provide health information prior to discharge, some patients deny that they have been given any information on the day of surgery (Oberle et al., 1994). Similarly, information given to the patient at pre-assessment prior to admission may be forgotten, because at this early stage motivation is low and any information learned may not be retained (Oberle et al., 1994). In addition, the unfamiliar ward environment and fear of impending surgery at the time of pre-assessment may cause an increase in anxiety (Oberle et al., 1994), which in turn may cause poor retention of information provided (Kempe & Gelazis, 1985).

Clearly, reinforcing patient education and providing educational support following day surgery are factors essential to a patient's post-operative recovery, and a telephone call within 24 hours of discharge is a valid method of providing the patient with the additional post-operative support required. Nurses also appear to benefit from providing a follow-up telephone call. Fallo (1991) identified that nurses increased their self-esteem and benefited from improved staff morale as a result of providing the service. Burden (1992, p. 258) found that providing the continuity of care served to increase nurses' job satisfaction, and reported one nurse saying, 'I gain more than I give from the calls'.

The follow-up telephone call after day surgery has other functions as well. Burden (1992) identified that the follow-up telephone call can act to encourage a patient to comply with recommendations advised by the nursing staff, thus encouraging positive health behaviour. Furthermore, comments made by the patient during the telephone call can be recorded and used in improving subsequent patient care, thus serving as a part of the unit's quality assurance programme (Carrington, 1993). The follow-up telephone call can have a positive effect on a unit's marketing strategy, as the follow-up contact can reinforce the quality of care provided by the unit to potential purchasers of the service (Burden, 1992). Finally, the follow-up telephone call can be used as a method for directly evaluating patient satisfaction with the day surgical unit. Patients can voice any compliments or complaints to the nurse making the telephone call (Burden, 1992), and satisfaction can be measured. As satisfaction is 'continually at the forefront of change' (James, 1993, p. 23), the unit can identify the positive and negative dimensions of the service through patients' evaluations, and subsequently act to improve its services (Gunter-Hunt et al., 1982).

Mobile phone link

A recent development in some units, is for day surgery nurses to be 'on call' to their patients following discharge through a mobile telephone line. After discharge, patients are given the opportunity of asking a day surgery nurse for advice by telephone if post-operative complications arise prior to midnight following the day of their operation. The nurse holding the mobile telephone is paid to be 'on call'. She or he needs to be experienced in day surgery, and able to advise patients on what action to take if problems arise. If necessary the nurses are able to telephone on-call medical staff for advice or to expedite admission bypassing the accident and emergency department.

Conclusion

As most post-operative management is undertaken by the patient and his or her relatives at home, it is vital that the patient is fully prepared for early discharge from the day surgical unit. Day surgery offers the patient total care, and as the prime care provider, the nurse plays a crucial role in helping to guide the patient towards self-care. By using the framework of a care plan for guidance, the nurse can assess, plan, implement and evaluate the patient care delivered. The nurse is also able to guide and assist patients towards meeting their own self-care needs.

By following discharge policies the nurse assures the patient's safety on discharge from the unit, and by setting up support mechanisms the nurse enables the patient to be confident with early discharge and able to seek assistance if required.

References

Audit Commission (1991a) A Shortcut to Better Services. London: HMSO.

Audit Commission (1991b) Measuring Quality – The Patients' View of Day Surgery. London: HMSO.

Avis M (1992) Silent partners. British Journal of Theatre Nursing October 2(7): 8–11.

Bailey JM (1993) Day surgery; a problem of economics or financial management? Ambulatory Surgery 1(3): 125–128.

Bowling A (1993) Assessing health needs and measuring patient satisfaction. Nursing Times 88(31): 31–34.

Bridger P, Rees M (1995) What a difference a day makes. Health Service Journal 20 April 105(5449): 22–23.

Burden N (1992) Telephone follow-up of ambulatory patients following discharge is a nursing responsibility. Journal of Post-Anaesthesia Nursing 7(4): 256–261.

Bysshe JE (1988) The effect of giving information to patients before surgery. Nursing 30: 36–39.

Caldwell L (1991) The influence of preference for information on preoperative stress and coping in surgical outpatients. Applied Nursing Research 4(4): 177–183.

Carrington S (1993) Day surgery in Bristol. British Journal of Theatre Nursing February 3(2): 12–15.

Dale F (1993) Postoperative pain in the elective surgical patient. British Journal of Nursing 2(17): 842–849.

Davies PRF, Ogg TW (1993) Managing anaesthesia for geriatric day surgery. Journal of One Day Surgery 2(4): 16–18.

Dobree L (1989) Pre-admission booklets for patients awaiting surgery. Nursing Times 85(4): 42–44.

Dutton KEA (1994) Patient education in a day surgery unit. Journal of One Day Surgery 3(4): 22–24.

Fallo PC (1991) Developing a programme to monitor patient satisfaction and outcome in the ambulatory surgery setting. Journal of Post-Anasesthesia Nursing 6(3): 176–180.

Farquharson M (1993) Day surgery for patients over 70 years old. Journal of One Day Surgery 3(1): 20–21.

Farrelly H, Lakeman D (1994) Patient education in day care. Journal of One Day Surgery 3(3): 18–20.

Gunter-Hunt G, Ferguson KJ, Bole GG (1982) Appointment keeping behaviour and patient satisfaction: implication for health professionals. Patient Counselling & Health Education 3(4): 156–160.

Haines N (1992) Same day surgery. AORN Journal 55(2): 573–580.

Haines M, Viellion G (1990) A successful combination: preadmission testing and preoperative education. Orthopaedic Nursing 9(2): 53–57.

Henderson V (1988) Patient education and literature review. Journal of Advanced Nursing 13: 203–213.

Hodge D (1993) Nurse specialisation in day surgery. Journal of One Day Surgery 3(1): 19.

Hodge D (1994) Introduction to day surgery. Surgical Nurse 7(2): 12–16.

Jackson IJB, Blackburn A, Tams J, Thirlway M (1993) Expansion of day surgery. A survey of general practitioners' views. Journal of One Day Surgery 2(4): 4–7.

James R (1993) Night and day. Health Service Journal 103(5367): 22–24.

Kempe AR (1987) Ambulatory surgery. AORN Journal 45(2): 500–507.

Kempe AR, Gelazis R (1985) Patient anxiety levels. AORN Journal 41(2): 390–396.

Markanday L, Platzer H (1994) Brief encounters. Nursing Times 90(70): 38–42.

Medical Defence Union (1992) Risk management in day surgery. Journal of One Day Surgery June 2(1): 8–9.

Mitchell M (1994) Pre-operative and post-operative psychological nursing care. Surgical Nurse 7(3): 22–25.

NHS Executive (1994) Day Surgery Task Force Report (Update). London: HMSO.

NHSME (1991) Day Surgery – Making it Happen. London: HMSO.

NHSME (1993) Day Surgery Taskforce Report. London: HMSO.

Oberle K, Allen M, Lynkowski P (1994) Follow-up of same day surgery patients. AORN Journal 59(5): 1016–1025.

Orem D (1991) Nursing Concepts of Practice. St Louis: Mosby.

Penn S (1993) Education in day surgery: a nursing view. Journal of One Day Surgery 3(2): 10–11.

Ralphs D (1994) Is day surgery for you? British Journal of Theatre Nursing 4(1): 4–8.

Reynolds A, Morgan M (1991) Day-to-day image problems. Health Service Journal 15 August 2(7): 18–19.

Rickford F, Lyall J (1995) Welcome words. Health Service Journal 16 February 101: 5–6.

Royal College of Surgeons (1985) Guidelines of Day Care Surgery. London: Royal College of Surgeons.

Royal College of Surgeons (1992) Guidelines for Day Surgery. London: Royal College of Surgeons.

Ruckley CV, Garraway WM, Cuthbertson C, Fenwick N, Prescott RJ (1980) The community nurse and day surgery. Nursing Times 76(6): 255–256.

Salmon P (1993) The reduction of anxiety in surgical patients: an important nursing task or the medicalization of preparatory worry? International Journal of Nursing Studies 30(4): 323–330.

Seers K (1987) Perceptions of pain. Nursing Times 83(48): 37–39.

Senapati A, Young AE (1989) Acceptability of day case surgery. Journal of the Royal Society of Medicine 82: 735–736.

Sutherland R (1994) Is this the way forward? British Journal of Theatre Nursing 4(1): 12–13.

UKCC (1992a) The Scope of Professional Practice. London: UKCC.

UKCC (1992b) The Code of Professional Conduct. London: UKCC.

Vasquez MA (1992) From theory to practice: Orem's self-care nursing model and ambulatory care. Journal of Post-Anaesthesia Nursing 7(4): 251–255.

Young CM (1990) The post-operative follow-up phone call; an essential part of the ambulatory surgery nurse's job. Journal of Post-Anaesthesia Nursing 5(4): 273–275.

Further reading

Alderman C (1990) Day tripper. Nursing Standard 4(40): 22–23.

Black N, Petticrew M, Hunter D, Sanderson C (1993) Day surgery: development of a national comparative audit service. Quality in Health Care 2: 162–166.

Boyce J (1993) Ambulatory surgery in the UK Ambulatory Surgery 1(3): 129–131.

Bradshaw C, Pritchett C, Eccles M, Armitage T, Wright H, Todd E (1987) South Tyneside fasttrack day surgery planning. Journal of One Day Surgery 34(4): 6–8.

Burn JMB (1979) A blueprint for day surgery. Anaesthesia 43: 790–805.

Buttery Y, Sissons J, Williams KN (1993) Patients' views one week after day surgery with general anaesthesia. Journal of One Day Surgery 3(1): 6–8.

Carrington S (1993) Quality assurance in day surgery. Journal of One Day Surgery 2(3): 15–19.

Chapman P (1991) It's better by day. Health Service Journal 19 September: 18–20.

Gay S, Bradshaw K, O'Bourke T, Chuan Y, Probert C, Mayberry J (1993) Patients' satisfaction survey. Journal of Royal Society of Health 113(3): 121–123.

Ghosh S (1994) Are the Audit Commission's targets realistic? Journal of One Day Surgery 4(2): 19–21.

Ghosh S, Kershaw AR (1991) The patients' and general practitioners' notions of day surgery. Journal of One Day Surgery 1(3): 10–11.

Ghosh S, Sallam S (1994) Patient satisfaction and post-operative demands on hospital and community services after day surgery. British Journal of Surgery 81(11): 1635–1638.

Grainger C, Griffiths R (1993) Over the obstacles. Health Service Journal 103(5349): 24-25.

Hagopian GA, Rubenstein H (1990) Effects of telephone call interventions on patients' wellbeing in a radiation therapy dept. Cancer Nursing 13(6): 339–344.

Hardie RM (1993) Day surgery assessement nurse. Journal of One Day Surgery 2(3):19–20.

Hawkshaw D (1994) A day surgery patient telephone follow-up survey. British Journal of Nursing 3(7): 348–350.

Hind M, Mason J (1994) Professional and managerial issues in day surgery. British Journal of Theatre Nursing 4(1): 17.

Icenhour ML (1988) Quality interpersonal care. AORN Journal 47(6): 1414–1419.

Lepczyk M, Raleigh EH, Rowley C (1990) Timing of preoperative patient teaching. Journal of Advanced Nursing 15: 300–306.

Lyall J (1995) Gains and pains. Health Service Journal 16 February: 1–2.

MacKenzie-Page S, Laurel A, Beresford LA (1988) Planning and documentation. AORN Journal 47(2): 526–537.

Meaden S (1993) The achievement of day care staff rotation. Journal of One Day Surgery 3(3): 21–24.

Meredith P, Wood C (1994) The introduction of an audit programme to measure patient satisfaction with surgical care. Journal of One Day Surgery 4(2): 15–16.

Morgan M, Beech R (1990) Variations in length of stay and rates of day case surgery. Journal of Epidemiology & Community Health 44: 90–103.

Noon BE, Davero CC (1987) Patient satisfaction in a hospital based day surgery setting. AORN Journal 46(2): 306–311.

Paton A (1990) Day surgery – satisfaction and savings. THS Health Summary 7(12): 5.

Robinson R (1994) Day shift. Health Service Journal 104(5390): 28–29.

Sandison AJP, Jones SE, Jones PA (1994) A daycare modified shouldice hernia repair follow-up. Journal of One Day Surgery 3(4): 16–17.

Chapter 7
Care of children in the day surgical unit

Sharon Bole

Introduction

This chapter looks at children and day surgery. It examines the special needs of children and discusses whether these needs can be met within an adult day surgical unit (DSU). It considers the specialist facilities and skills needed to ensure a high standard of care, and looks at what can be done to alleviate the stresses associated with day surgery for both children and their carers.

The Platt report (1959) on the welfare of children in hospital was an important government report into the arrangements made for children in hospital – aside from their medical treatment. It recognised the child as an individual and the importance of the family unit. Among its recommendations were those that children and adolescents should not be nursed in adult wards but in the company of other children of similar age, that they should have facilities for play and that their surroundings should be cheerful and safe.

These recommendations are still as relevant today as they were in 1959, although being only recommendations they are not always implemented. Children are naturally more relaxed in their own home environment, where they can play with their own toys and sleep in their own beds. However, children still require surgery and despite many technical advances we have not yet progressed to taking the operating theatre out into private homes. Day surgery would seem to be the next best option – children are only admitted to hospital for a day, sometimes only half a day, to have their operation, and are then allowed back home to be cared for by their parents.

There are, however, many issues to be considered before we can be sure that we are providing safe, high quality care for these children and their families. Firstly, it is necessary to define a child in a day surgery context. A telephone survey of five DSUs by the author found that most accepted children between the ages of 1 and 12 years. Those under one year tend to be more of an anaesthetic risk than older children and are more often dealt with as in-patients. Those over 12 fall into the category of adolescents and, ideally, should be nursed with others of the same age in separate facilities. In practice, it is unlikely that many DSUs will have dedicated adolescent facilities, more likely each patient will be individually assessed and then offered accommodation in either the adult ward, a side room, or in the paediatric area, whichever seems most appropriate.

What are the special needs of children and can they be met within an adult day surgical unit?

Children are a unique group of patients. Children of all ages have special, individual health care needs. They are physically, psychologically and emotionally different from adults.

A basic knowledge of child developmental psychology is needed to understand the way children think, their behaviour and their reactions. Swiss scientist Jean Piaget, cited in Duncombe & Weller (1979), described several stages of a child's cognitive development, and these stages can be used to help us understand a child's thinking and reactions to being in hospital. Piaget said that by the age of one year a child has developed a strong bond with his or her mother and knows she still exists even if he or she cannot see her. A child of this age is more likely to cry for his or her mother than a younger child. Children at this stage are still too young to understand explanations or reasoning and are best communicated with through their parents.

A pre-school child is defenceless and immature in both body and mind. He or she has not yet learned to express him or herself clearly or to be adaptable, and needs the security of his or her usual routine, familiar surroundings and familiar faces. Emotionally the pre-school child is still immature, incapable of understanding 'tomorrow' and lives only in the present. He or she has a lively imagination and easily twists what he or she sees and hears into frightening fantasies. A pre-school child is sensitive to the tone of people's voices, to their expressions and gestures, and is easily alarmed. At this stage it is the mother who not only interprets the surroundings for her child but acts as a buffer between the child and his or her surroundings (Duncombe & Weller, 1979)

Piaget's second stage, age two to seven years, is a very egocentric stage with everything revolving around the child, such as 'I am ill because I was naughty'. The most striking aspects of hospital to children of this age are likely to be material, such as lights in operating theatres, visible wounds, blood, uniforms and strange beds. Children under the age of seven are unable to see the relationship between treatment and cure, and are likely to see any painful treatment as punishment for being naughty.

Children aged 7–12 years are less egocentric and more logical. They are able to see a relationship between illness and its treatment and are able to understand that treatment is intended to help them, although they are still only able to relate to concrete objects and things that they have actually experienced. Above the age of 12 children are able to think abstractly; they can imagine, reason and symbolise (Brunner & Suddarth, 1991)

It is not possible to state a chronological age at which adolescence begins. It is commonly thought to start when a child reaches his or her teens but it is a variable event related to the maturity of the child. For some it may start as early as 10 years of age, for others not until 14 years and it may continue until 21 years of age.

Adolescence is a time of great change – emotionally, physically, sexually, socially and culturally. All areas are evolving and maturing. An adolescent is becoming an individual in his or her own right, leaving childhood behind and moving towards adulthood. He or she is striving for independence and to develop his or her own identify, and will fight fiercely to defend this. Adolescents need to feel that they have a say in what is happening to them. They expect honest, accurate information and easily distrust anyone who is less then honest with them. Most adolescents would see themselves as too old to be nursed with children but many feel uncomfortable when nursed with adults (Muller et al., 1992).

This brief insight into a child's thinking shows how different children are from adults and from each other. Children do not all develop at the same speed and a room full of six-year-olds may all be at different stages of cognitive development. Because children are not always able to express what they are feeling or what they need, it is important that they have people around them who are able to interpret for them. Outside of hospital it is their parents and families who do this for them. In hospital it is not always possible for their parents to continue this role in all areas. This may be because some hospitals do not allow parents to accompany their children at all times, for example in the recovery room or because the situation itself is too stressful or beyond the parents' understanding.

The Platt report (1959) recommended that children should be cared for by a nurse with child developmental knowledge, with a recognised children's nursing qualification and with experience in the care of children. The Department of Health in its 1991 report into the welfare of children in hospital recognised the specialist skills required to look after a sick child safely and set target standards – that there should be at least two registered sick children's nurses (or project 2000 child branch) on duty in all children's wards and departments where children are cared for, and that a registered sick children's nurse should be on duty in other areas to advise on the care of children. Unfortunately, these are only recommendations and not compulsory requirements and even if they were, the current nationwide shortage of paediatric nurses would make them unworkable.

It is unlikely that most DSUs will have a paediatric nurse on their staff. Good links with nurses on the paediatric ward will prove invaluable to help guide day surgery nurses involved in the care of children. The philosophy of care for nursing children should be family centred. Children cannot be nursed in isolation, and it is important to recognise that the family is the centre of a child's life and that all the care given should be aimed at supporting and strengthening the competence of that family to care for their child.

The 1993 Audit Commission report *Children First* looked at the provision and quality of hospital services for children and stressed that the specialist needs of children and their families could not be met without staff who have skills to deal with children and to provide care and support for the whole family. This is particularly important in the day surgery scenario where it is the family who will be responsible for the ongoing care of their child following discharge.

Each family is individual with its own structure and background creating its own strengths, weaknesses and needs. It is important to respect a family's racial, ethnic, cultural and socio-economic variants and to recognise different methods of coping. Nursing care should be given in a supportive and unbiased manner. Care of the child should be a collaboration between parents and hospital staff, a partnership enabling parents to maintain a sense of participation and control, supported by hospital staff.

In addition to recommendations for nursing staff there are also recommendations for medical staff and suitable day surgery operations. The Audit Commission report (1993) cites the National Confidential Enquiry into peri-operative deaths as saying '... surgeons and anaesthetists should not undertake occasional paediatric practice. The outcome of surgery is related to the experience of the clinicians involved'. The enquiry found that in a sample of 1000 surgeons and 2000 anaesthetists, 87 per cent of surgeons said that they operated on children, but 24 per cent of them did fewer than 20 such operations per year. Similarly 15 per cent of anaesthetists said that they anaesthetised fewer than 20 children aged 3–10 years per year.

The British Association of Paediatric Surgeons in its 1994 report *A Guide For Purchasers of Paediatric Surgical Services* recommended that a general surgeon providing non-specialist paediatric surgery should:

- have had six months' training in paediatric surgery;
- care for a sufficient number of children each year to maintain a high level of competence;
- have at least one operating list per week dedicated to children;
- maintain continuing education in paediatric surgery.

The Royal College of Surgeons of England in its *Guidelines for Day Case Surgery* (1992) published a comprehensive list of suitable operations for day case surgery in children. Some examples are given in Figure 7.1. Lists are not static and change constantly in line with developments and experience.

Special facilities needed

Toys

The facilities provided for children and their families within an adult DSU need special consideration. Children arriving for elective day surgery are generally fit and healthy and are unlikely to stay on their bed or trolley during the early part of their admission, therefore, facilities for play must be available. Play is a universal way of communicating for children. We can learn a lot about a child through play as they lose their inhibitions and show more of their inner self while involved in their activities.

Giving a child a variety of play materials provides the opportunity for spontaneous play. By limiting the materials available we can use directed play to focus on a specific area, for example using medical equipment to explore a fear of injections or to play out aspects of the operation that a child is about to have, or to prepare a child for a specific procedure. Play provides a familiar means of relaxation and

General/Urology

Inguinal hernia
Umbilical hernia
Epigastric hernia
Hydrocele
Orchidopexy
Circumcision
Sigmoidoscopy
Examination under anaesthetic
Division of preputial adhesions
Excision of skin lesions

Orthopaedic

Manipulation under anaesthetic
Change of plaster
Removal of pins/plates/screws
Trigger thumb
Arthroscopy

ENT

Removal of foreign bodies
Examination under anaesthetic
Dewax and suction clearance
Tympanoplasty
Release of tongue tie
Adenoidectomy
Tonsillectomy
Myringotomy and grommets
Submucosal resection
Submucosal diathermy

Ophthalmic

Syringe and probing
Strabismus correction (squint)
Examination under anaesthetic
Chalazion and other cysts

Plastic surgery

Bat ears correction
Dermoid cyst excision
Simple/incomplete syndactyly
Excision of accessory digits/auricles

Figure 7.1: Operations suitable for day case surgery in children

diversion, helping the child to feel more secure in a new and strange environment. It allows them to express their feelings, reduces anxiety and releases tension. Allowing a child to play with miniature or actual equipment or encouraging children to play out an experience before a procedure may help to work out any misconceptions or fears.

Toys should be good quality and suitable for a range of ages and abilities. They should be interesting and safe, and it is important to remember that what is safe for one age-group may not be safe for another. Younger children, particularly those under three years, still tend to put things into their mouths. It is important, therefore, to avoid any toys with small parts, which may be aspirated, swallowed or may choke the child. Packaging on toys usually recommends a specific age-group suitability.

Toys also need to be robust enough to withstand rough play. Children love to explore toys, to see how they are made and will always try to pull a toy apart. Look for sturdy construction, check that eyes and noses are tightly secured to soft toys and conform to safety standards. Materials should be non-toxic and, where appropriate, flame retardant. Toys should be inspected regularly for loose or broken parts checking for potential hazards.

Toys suitable for older children should be stored on higher shelves out of reach of youngsters. A hospital play specialist, usually linked to the paediatric ward will be able to give invaluable help in deciding the suitability and storage of toys.

Safety

The general environment of the unit should be made as friendly as possible and designed with children in mind. Safety is paramount; childproof fittings, high door handles to restrict access to potentially dangerous areas, reducing the temperature of hot tap water to prevent scalding and covering electric plug sockets are some of the considerations to reduce the likelihood of danger to curious, active children.

Trolley sides should be long enough to prevent a child from falling off at either end of the trolley and the spacing between the bars should be narrow enough to prevent a child's head from getting stuck between them. Removable padded cot-sides prevent restless children from knocking themselves on the trolley as they are waking from anaesthesia. Curtains or screens should be available for privacy as children can be just as shy or self-conscious as adults.

Facilities for parents

Facilities for parents are equally as important. There should be comfortable chairs available for them while they sit with their child as he or she is recovering. Parents are often reluctant to leave the unit in case their child should need them, so tea and coffee facilities should be available for parents and visitors. Parents often choose not to eat or drink in front of their fasting child before coming in for day surgery, and they should be encouraged to have something to eat or drink while waiting for their child to return from the operating theatre.

Parents may want to make telephone calls to other family members or to arrange transport home; an easily accessible public telephone is important so that parents do not have to leave their child for long periods. There should be a direct line telephone number to enable parents to contact the unit if they have any problems or queries after their child is discharged home. Some units also provide an out of hours service with a senior nurse carrying a mobile phone to provide advice if required.

Anaesthesia

As well as the emotional and psychological differences already discussed, children present special, individual physical differences. From an anaesthetic point of view most problems are likely to occur in children under three years of age. Anaesthesia in an older child is very similar to that of an adult. The structure and development of the chest and lungs in the younger child means that they are less able to sustain increased respiratory effort. During infancy the lungs are still developing – the lumen of the trachea and bronchi are relatively small in comparison with the volume of the lung, giving high resistance to inspired air. Small airways are easily blocked by oedema and mucus. There is a relatively large amount of dead space within the respiratory system, which means that the infant must breathe twice as fast as an adult to supply the body with the necessary oxygen.

A child's larynx is narrowest at the cricoid cartilage, and pressure from an endotracheal tube may cause oedema, which obstructs air flow after extubation. A child also has a relatively large tongue, which may make intubation more difficult. Children under six months of age have an immature swallowing reflex and may have gastro-oesophageal reflux which increases the risk of aspiration under anaesthetic (Mackay, 1996).

Upper respiratory tract infections are very common in the paediatric population and as it is not recommended to anaesthetise an ill child unless it is unavoidable, this means that elective, i.e. non-emergency, cases are often cancelled. Multiple cancellations can create scheduling problems for families and emotional problems for children, not to mention disruption to theatre lists.

Studies have shown an increased risk of cough, laryngospasm, pneumonia and hypoxia when children with an upper respiratory tract infection (URTI) undergo anaesthesia. However, it is important to remember that there are children who may appear to have an URTI but who may actually have a chronic or other non-infectious condition. Distinguishing between the different conditions is not always easy. Tait and Knight (1987) have developed a set of criteria to help identify symptoms which qualify as an URTI. A combination of two of the following (except as in 8) qualifies as an URTI:

1. sore or scratchy throat;
2. sneezing;
3. rhinorrhoea;
4. congestion;
5   malaise;
6. non-productive cough;
7. low grade pyrexia;
8. combinations of 1 + 5, 2 + 3, 3 + 6, or 4 + 6 require an additional symptom for diagnosis.

The history and physical examination may also be helpful. Other family members may have symptoms or may have just recovered from them. An apyrexial child with a clear nasal discharge most likely has an allergic rhinitis. The presence of grunting, nasal flaring, or use of accessory respiratory muscles suggests lower respiratory involvement. Wheezing, for whatever reason, is enough to cancel an elective operation.

If surgery needs to be postponed the ideal timing for rescheduling appears to be a minimum of six weeks after symptoms of lower respiratory tract infection and two to four weeks after the last symptoms of an URTI (Tait & Knight, 1987).

Observations

When looking after anxious, frightened children even simple tasks such as taking a child's pulse, temperature and blood pressure can become a difficult, skilled task. Infants do not have an easily palpable radial pulse and are unlikely to keep their hand and arm still to allow you to try. By far the easiest method is to use a stethoscope to record the apex beat, and allowing the child to listen to their own heart first often makes them more co-operative. Other sites for palpating a pulse include temporal, brachial, femoral and pedal pulses.

A variety of devices are available for taking a child's temperature. The traditional glass mercury thermometer is perhaps the most well known, but probably the least safe for use with children. Glass is breakable and mercury is toxic; it is important to have a child's co-operation when using this device. The child must be able to breathe through his or her nose and close his or her mouth without biting, and to keep still for the desired length of time – usually impossible for most under-fives. The same thermometer can be used to record an axillary temperature. Although this is generally accepted as less accurate than the oral or rectal route it is safer. Rectal temperature recording is no longer commonly used. It is an undignified, insulting procedure for the child and the risk of perforating the rectum is greatly increased by the child moving.

There are various other temperature-recording devices on the market, many of which have advantages for paediatric patients. The electronic thermometer has a metal probe with an unbreakable plastic sheath; it can be used orally, axillary or rectally and registers temperature within 60 seconds. The tympanic membrane sensor gives an extremely accurate reading. It is quick, giving a digital display within 1–2 seconds. It is recommended that three measurements are taken and the highest recorded. Plastic strip thermometers, such as those placed on the forehead, have variable accuracy and are best used for screening children for pyrexia rather than for an accurate measurement. They are convenient and easy to use for parents at home. Disposable, single-use thermometers, such as Tempa Dot, produce a chemical reaction which causes dots to change colour. They have been found to be fairly accurate, easy to read and are much safer than glass (Whaley & Wong, 1995).

Temperature regulation can be a problem in children, particularly younger children. Children have a large surface area compared with their body mass and quickly lose heat, particularly from their heads. This is important to remember when the child is exposed during surgery. Whenever possible, the head and limbs should be covered to reduce heat loss. An electric warming pad may be placed on the theatre table to help maintain the child's temperature.

Routine checking of a child's blood pressure is an important way of screening for congenital renal or cardiac anomalies. As with adults, an accurate recording depends on having the correct size cuff. It must be wide enough to cover 75 per cent of the upper arm and long enough to encircle the limb completely with or without an overlap. A cuff that is too small will give a falsely high blood pressure reading, one that is too large will give a falsely low reading. Normal blood pressure in children is variable with the age and size of the child. For example, in two children of the same age but with one larger and taller than the other, the larger child will have a higher normal blood pressure than the smaller child. Average normal blood pressures are approximately:

- newborn: 65/40;
- 1 month–2 years: 95/58;
- 2–5 years: 100/57 (Whaley & Wong, 1995).

Children easily become anxious which may elevate their blood pressure. Explaining each step of the procedure will help to gain their co-operation and reduce anxiety. Allowing them to handle the equipment or turning the procedure into a game, such as pretending to test the strength of the child's muscles and getting them to watch how high the silver line goes up, also helps children to relax. Play is a universal language for children, and bringing play into any procedure can help a child to relax and co-operate.

Pre-operative fasting

For many years, one of the major potential anaesthetic risks was aspiration of gastric contents into the lungs. The usual approach to prevent this was a prolonged period of fasting to ensure 'an empty stomach'. Typically this has been four hours in newborns and young infants and six hours in older children. Unfortunately this meant that these children began surgery with a fluid deficit, they were irritable because they were hungry and thirsty, and parents, who were already stressed and anxious, became more distressed as they were unable to console their miserable child. Occasionally surgery had to be cancelled due to inadvertent eating or drinking during the fasting period.

Parents are usually given instructions to fast their child from midnight. But because young children often have their last food or drink before going to bed at around 7pm and parents are reluctant to wake them, when admitted to a DSU at 8am the child may have been fasted for between 12 and 13 hours. Fortunately, several recent studies in children have shown that a fast of only two to three hours after clear fluids is all that is needed (solids and other fluids are withheld for six hours prior to surgery); residual gastric volumes were equal to or less than those undergoing a protracted fast (Cote, 1990; Dershewitz, 1993).

Relieving stress

A lot can be done to prepare a child for his or her admission to hospital. The aims are to make the unit less strange and frightening both to the child and his or her parents; to familiarise them with the routine they will experience on the day; to provide the opportunity for children and parents to see the unit, including the operating theatre and recovery; and to allow them to see and touch some of the equipment that they will see on the day of surgery. Parents should be given the opportunity to ask questions without their child being present and the child should also have the opportunity to ask questions.

Preparation sessions should be planned before the child's admission to hospital, often this is done on a Saturday as it may enable both parents and siblings to take part as well. Group sessions must take into account each child's individual needs, including developmental needs and variable previous experiences. Group sizes should be small enough to be manageable and to allow discussion. Small children have a limited retentive memory so their visits need to be arranged for about two to three weeks before the expected date of admission. A prepared slide show, video or film can be used to tell the story of a child during a day surgery operation day, from admission to discharge.

Opportunities for dressing up in theatre hats, masks and gowns, and playing with stethoscopes, syringes and bandages allows children to play out their fantasies and allows staff to correct any misconceptions the child may have. A ride on a theatre trolley or wheelchair can add an element of fun while familiarising children with hospital equipment.

Honesty is important; not mentioning something because it may be frightening will not help to prepare the child for the event. The unexpected or the unknown are more upsetting and stressful than threats that are known, and a child's fantasies are often more scary than reality. Young children are very egocentric and perceive everything as relating to them, so procedures and events should be described in terms of what they will actually see, hear, taste, smell and feel. Emphasising areas where the child can help will enable them to feel that they still have some control over what is going on. Preparing children not only decreases their anxiety but can help to promote their co-operation.

It is important to allow the child time to feel relaxed in his or her new surroundings, allowing a short time for play will give him or her time to settle in. Don't rush up to the child, grinning broadly, talking loudly and staring them hard in the eye, this may seem threatening or intimidating. Talk to the parents initially if the child is shy, they will soon become curious, they will watch you and will eventually want to be part of the conversation. It may be useful to use a favourite toy, such as a doll, teddy or puppet, talking to the toy rather than directly to the child. Whenever possible you should position yourself at eye level with the child – it is much less threatening than having a stranger towering above you asking questions.

During a child's admission the greatest amount of verbal communication will be with the parents, but it is important not to exclude the child from the conversation. Children are very alert, they can attach meaning to every gesture and move that you make, particularly younger children. Speaking in a quiet, unhurried manner is calming, being confident and positive in your attitude is reassuring. Use language that the child can understand, with simple words and short sentences. Children should be given time to ask their own questions. Take their concerns and fears seriously and give older children the opportunity to talk without their parents being present.

If the opportunity arises give the child the chance to make choices in his or her own treatment, for example gaseous or intravenous induction of anaesthetic. The Children Act (Department of Health, 1989) and the Children's Charter (Department of Health, 1996) promote the rights of the child to have a say in his or her care. Once the child is old enough chronologically and mentally to make an informed decision he or she can refuse to submit to a procedure. It is the job of nursing and medical staff to make sure that both parents and children are given the necessary information to make an informed choice. Once a child is capable of making his or her own decision the rights of the parents may have to yield to those of the child. This holds great implications for obtaining consent for surgery, and for giving injections, suppositories or other procedures where the child should be consulted beforehand.

Analgesia

Good analgesia is important in the care of children. Unfortunately health professionals tend to underestimate the amount of pain that children experience. Pain is a personal experience and each child's pain is whatever that child says it is. It is important that children are believed when they say they have pain, whether the pain is expressed verbally or non-verbally. Children are often undertreated for pain because of a number of fallacies about paediatric pain control. The two most common of these are fear of respiratory depression and fear of addiction. However, narcotics are no more dangerous for children than they are for adults. Addiction to opioids used for analgesia is extremely rare in children.

Adequate pain relief is a basic need of all patients, and children are no exception. They have the right to receive the right drug at the right dose by the right route at the right time. Although nurses do not prescribe analgesia it is important that they are aware of correct dosages and possible side effects. The optimum dose is one that controls pain without causing severe side effects.

It is useful to have a specialist paediatric drug dosage book available, as adult books tend only to give generalised references for children. Children's dosages are calculated according to their body weight not their age. All nurses involved in the care of children should be able to calculate the correct dose of drugs for the children in their care. It is a nurse's responsibility to ensure that the drugs they give are within safe and effective dosage limits. Nurses not regularly involved in the care of children may not be familiar with paediatric drug dosages and should always check before administering any medication to children, and should not be afraid to question dosages that seem incorrect. The United Kingdom Central Council Code of Professional Conduct states that nurses must safeguard and promote the interests of their patients, must ensure that no action or omission is detrimental to their patients and must acknowledge any limitations in knowledge or competence (UKCC, 1992). An example of the calculation of the correct paracetamol dosage for a child weighing 24 kg is given in Figure 7.2.

Recommended dosage (oral or rectal) is 10–15 mg per kg per dose, therefore dosage would be:

@ 10mg/kg   24kg × 10mg/kg = 240mg per dose, minimum therapeutic dosage

@ 15mg/kg   24kg × 15mg/kg = 360mg per dose, maximum therapeutic dosage

Figure 7.2: Calculation of the correct paracetamol dosage for a child weighing **24 kg** (Royal Liverpool Childrens Hospital, 1994)

It is not unusual for medical staff to be very cautious when prescribing analgesia for children, writing 5 ml of Calpol (= 120 mg paracetamol) for a child whose therapeutic dose is two to three times this. If you promise a child that taking the medicine will stop the pain, you should be sure that the dosage you are giving is sufficient to do this. A child will soon learn to distrust you if you do not keep your promises. A specialist paediatric drug dosage book, such as the *Alder Hey Book of Children's Doses*, produced by the Pharmacy Department of the Royal Liverpool Childrens Hospital (Alder Hey), is an invaluable reference.

A child who is in pain will not necessarily say so. Equally, a child sitting quietly may be doing so because it hurts to move. Young children may not know what the word 'pain' means, so it is important to use words appropriate to the child's age.

Children show various responses to pain. Young infants may become generally rigid or may thrash about, eyes closed, frowning and mouth open. Older infants will usually cry loudly with an expression of anger or pain. Young children will cry loudly or scream, will say 'ow' or 'ouch', and will thrash their arms and legs. They will cling to their mother or a nurse. They want a hug or other physical comfort. School-age children may clench their fists, grit their teeth, close their eyes and wrinkle their foreheads. A child's behaviour may indicate localised body pain, such as pulling at their ears for earache, rolling their head from side to side for headache and lying on their side with their legs drawn up for abdominal pain.

A pain rating scale is a useful tool to assess the amount of pain that a child is experiencing. Children as young as three are able to use a faces pain rating scale as shown in Figure 7.3. It can be explained to the child that, for example, face 0 is very happy because he has no pain (hurt), face 1 hurts a little bit, face 2 hurts a little more and so on. Face 5 hurts as much as you can imagine, though you do not actually have to be crying to feel this bad. The child should be asked to choose the face that best describes how he or she is feeling.

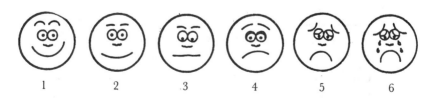

1   2   3   4   5   6

Figure 7.3: Pain rating scale suitable for use with young children
Reproduced by kind permission of Jim Richardson from 'Acute pain in childhood', Surgical Nurse (1992).

There are many routes and methods of giving analgesia to children suitable for day surgery use.

1. Oral (e.g. paracetamol, ibuprofen). This is a convenient method with a co-operative child, but it is impossible to make a child swallow something if he or she does not want to. Most drugs have a peak effect in one to two hours, therefore, it is not the route of choice for severe pain.

2. Intramuscular (e.g. codeine phosphate, pethidine). This is a painful route for administration and is hated by children. Some drugs cause pain at the injection site.

3. Rectal (e.g. paracetamol, Voltarol). This is an alternative to the oral route. It is generally disliked by children but preferred to the intramuscular route.

4. Regional block using a long-acting local anaesthetic, such as bupivacaine, injected into the site at the end of surgery, for example in hernia repair or penile block after circumcision.

5. Caudal. The use of caudal analgesia is increasingly being used following paediatric surgery, such as circumcision. A quantity of local anaesthetic is injected into the caudal space causing sensory and often motor blockade to the area supplied by the nerves around and below the injection point. Anatomical changes with age make this procedure easier and the spread of analgesia more predictable in children under the age of seven years. The quality of sensory block is influenced by the choice and quantity of local anaesthetic used. Best results appear to be achieved by using 0.25per cent bupivicaine, 0.75 per kg, giving a sensory block lasting up to five hours. A retrospective study of 750 children undergoing caudal blocks between October 1982 and December 1987 at the Hotel-Dieu Hospital, France, showed a 96 per cent success rate, that is, a good, symmetrical sensory block with or without motor blockade. However, this procedure is not without side effects. Patients with motor blockade were found to be more restless post-operatively than those without, and nausea and vomiting were not uncommon, occurring in approximately 17 per cent of those studied. Five per cent developed pruritus, two per cent pyrexia and one per cent skin rashes. First voiding may be delayed following caudal analgesia, but no patient in the study required

bladder catheterisation. Overall this is a safe, acceptable method of analgesia for children, particularly those under seven years of age (Dalens & Hasnaoui, 1989).

Recovery

Care of a child in the recovery room is a skilled procedure and should not be undertaken without adequately qualified staff being available. Children should be nursed on a one to one basis until fully recovered. A child's condition may deteriorate rapidly and therefore needs skilled observation. Ideally, there should be a personal handover by the anaesthetist, with any special instructions being recorded on the anaesthetic chart. Routine recordings of pulse, respirations, blood pressure and pulse oximetry should be made.

A study of 16,700 consecutive paediatric patients in the recovery room at the Royal Manchester Children's Hospital from 1985–1988 showed that nearly all children show a drop in their blood pressure in recovery; over 30 per cent of children studied dropped their blood pressure by more than 33 per cent, compared with a drop of five per cent in most adults. Children tend to produce more nasopharyngeal secretions than adults and are often given atropine prior to or during anaesthesia to decrease these. Of those not receiving atropine, 23.8 per cent required suction (oropharyngeal); interestingly, only 0.85 per cent of these children developed any laryngospasm.

Anatomical differences in children mean that tasks such as the chin lift to maintain an open airway need to be performed in a different way to the way they are performed in adults. The degree of neck flexion should be minimal, as over-flexion can cause airway obstruction. When supporting the chin it is important that you only pull on the bony tip of the chin, as the floor of the mouth is easily compressed and if pressed may add to airway obstruction.

A child's heart has more conductive and connective tissue and less muscle than an adult's heart. Cardiac output is therefore more dependent on heart rate than on muscle contraction, and if bradycardia occurs it can be dangerous, causing lowered cardiac output. Deep nasotracheal suction should be avoided because vagal stimulation can cause bradycardia.

Each unit should have its own criteria for discharge from recovery. These may include:

•   able to maintain own airway;
•   able to move all four limbs;

- responds to verbal commands or speaks;
- able to lift head for four seconds.

In some DSUs children must be assessed by an anaesthetist before leaving recovery and returning to the ward, in others the anaesthetist devolves this responsibility to the nurses in the recovery room, providing they are experienced in the care of children and the anaesthetist has confidence in their ability.

Increasingly, parents are being allowed into the recovery area with their children. If this is to be the case there should be a dedicated paediatric recovery section and parents should be given clear guidelines of what to expect before entering recovery. Other criteria for allowing parents in recovery should include:

- the child should be awake;
- airway and cardiovascular stability is assured;
- no problems with any other patient in recovery;
- one parent per child;
- parent must agree to leave if asked (McConachie, Day & Morris, 1989).

However, if a child fulfils all the criteria it may be more suitable to return him or her to the ward area where the parents are waiting.

Criteria for discharging children following day surgery are similar to those for adults. Surgically, they should have fulfilled expected criteria for their specific operation, for example haemostatis, no excessive swelling, pain controlled. By far the most important criterion for discharging children following day surgery is that their parents must be happy and confident to take their children home.

Children usually manage to eat and drink soon after waking from anaesthetic. The best guide as to when they are ready is the child; a child asking for a drink or a biscuit is unlikely to be sick, whereas a child who is nauseated will be less willing to eat or drink. Parents and nursing staff should not push a child to eat or drink without taking time to find out why they are reluctant.

Waiting for a child to void post-operatively may prove to be a long process. After a prolonged fast it can be many hours before first voiding, particularly after caudal analgesia. As long as parents are made aware of the importance of watching for first voiding and know how to obtain help, it should not be necessary to keep a child in hospital until he or she has voided.

Ideally there should be two adults in the car to take a child home – one to drive and the other to supervise the child. Parents should be made aware that their child may exhibit some unusual behaviour following hospitalisation, such as aloofness towards his or her parents, being clingy, demanding attention, resisting separation, night waking, nightmares, temper tantrums and regression in newly learned skills (Whaley & Wong, 1995). These behaviours usually resolve themselves as the child settles back at home.

Parents should receive written information specific to their child's operation and generally about post-anaesthetic care. Clear, precise information about where to seek help or advice after day surgery is very important.

Conclusions

Children and their parents clearly present unique problems for nurses within a day surgery setting, but if staff are aware of these problems or potential problems, if they have good links with a paediatric ward to enable them to get help and advice whenever necessary and are committed to providing well informed, high quality care to these young patients who are not always able to speak for themselves, there should be no reason why children should not be safely accommodated within an adult DSU.

References

Alder Hey (1994) Alder Hey Book of Children's Doses, 6th edn. Pharmacy Office, Royal Liverpool Children's Hospital.

Audit Commission (1993) Children First – A study of Hospital Services. London: HMSO.

British Association of Paediatric Surgeons (1994) A Guide for Purchasers of Paediatric Surgical Services. Edinburgh: BAPS.

British Paediatric Association (1994) Welfare of Children and Young People in Hospital. London: BPA.

Brunner L, Suddarth D (1991) Lippincott Manual of Paediatric Nursing, 3rd edn. London: Chapman and Hall.

Cote CJ (1990) NPO after midnight - a reappraisal. Anaesthesiology 75.

Dalens B, Hasnaoui A (1989) Caudal anaesthesia in paediatric surgery. Anaesthetic Analgesia: 44.

Department of Health (1989) The Children Act – The Care of the Child. London: HMSO.

Department of Health (1991) Welfare of Children in Hospital. London: HMSO.

Department of Health (1996) The Patients' Charter – Services for Children and Young People. London: HMSO.

Dershewitz RA (1993) Ambulatory Paediatric Care, 2nd edn. Philadelphia: Lippincott.

Duncombe M, Weller B (1979) Paediatric Nursing. London: Baillière Tindall.

Mackay J (1996) From NATN Study Day. Little People. Paediatric Anaesthetics. Lecture.

McConachie I, Day A, Morris P (1989) Recovery from anaesthesia in children. Anaesthesia 44: 986–990.

Muller D, Harris P, Wattley L, Taylor J (1992) Nursing Children – Psychology, Research and Practice. London: Chapman and Hall.

Platt H (1959) The Welfare of Children in Hospital. London: HMSO.

Richardson J (1992) Acute pain in childhood. Surgical Nurse 5: 5.

Royal College of Surgeons (1992) Guidelines for Day Case Surgery. London: HMSO.

Tait AR, Knight PR (1987) The effects of general anaesthesia on upper respiratory tract infections in children. Anaesthesiology: 67.

United Kingdom Central Council for Nursing (1992) Midwifery and Health Visiting. Code of Professional Conduct. London: UKCC.

Whaley L, Wong DL (1995) Nursing Care of Infants and Children, 5th edn. St Louis: Mosby.

Chapter 8
Management of a day surgical unit

A brief introduction to management of a day surgical unit and the nurse's role

Louise Markanday

The role of the nurse, as we have seen, is multifaceted in terms of clinical skills. There is, however, another important role undertaken by the nurse: the role of manager or team leader. Nurses 'manage' in several ways. They organise and deliver care for their patients according to priority, and those with more experience take charge of a team of nurses as well as a caseload of patients. Nurses are often responsible for the day-to-day organisation of a day surgical unit (DSU). They ensure there are sufficient numbers of staff on duty, that levels of essential equipment are maintained and they take responsibility for the smooth and efficient running of the unit.

This chapter aims to provide an introduction to the management of a DSU for the nurse who takes charge occasionally or who is hoping for promotion. It briefly examines the role of more senior managers and offers some thoughts on how the physical environment affects the way in which day surgery care is delivered. It considers the advantages and disadvantages of 'stand-alone' units and provides a brief explanation of the recent NHS reforms and how these have affected day surgery care. The importance of audit is also discussed and explained.

The nurse in charge

The management of a ward or clinical area has traditionally been the domain of the ward sister or charge nurse. These highly skilled individuals commanded respect not only from their own staff but also from patients and medical staff. They ran the ward with almost military efficiency and were responsible for the clinical training of student and staff nurses, and they also held personal responsibility for the delivery of care to patients.

Nowadays, the ward sister is more often referred to as the 'ward manager' and frequently has responsibility for budget control, recruitment of staff and personnel issues, in addition to responsibility for the provision of safe, effective nursing care. Formerly, many of these functions were performed by the nursing officer and consequently, nurses have had to learn new skills to be able to fulfil the new demands of a ward manager's post. As these demands increase, staff nurses are also having to take on more managerial responsibility and the next section is aimed at those nurses who are adopting this role.

Staffing and its management

Nurses are by far the largest group of staff in a DSU and for this reason this section deals mainly with them, although the role of non-nursing staff is also examined. In recent years the status of the day surgery nurse has increased and she or he is now recognised as a knowledgeable, skilful practitioner who is able to perform several different functions within the unit. Many DSUs rotate nursing staff through the different areas of the unit with the effect of creating a multiskilled workforce. Sutherland (1994) fears that this will devalue nurses as they will not be experts in any one field. However, the author believes that nurses become day surgery experts with the necessary skills required for day surgery nursing; they are not partially skilled in theatre or ward nursing – a criticism often levelled at day surgery nurses by outsiders. Rotation of staff results in more interesting work for the nurse and a workforce that is flexible and can be moved about in times of need, such as staff sickness.

The skill of day surgery nursing is not merely 'ward', 'pre-assessment', 'theatre', 'anaesthetics' or 'recovery'. All five components make up the true day surgery practitioner who provides an holistic approach to care through understanding each process undergone by the patient. Day surgery nursing has an identity all of its own in the same way as intensive care or theatre nursing, and the rotation of staff has an important part to play in achieving this.

The intensiveness of day surgery nursing is often not appreciated by other nurses, who do not realise how much care, both physical and psychological, is delivered in a very short space of time. It is therefore a mistake to believe that a DSU can run efficiently and provide a high level of skilled care with only a few trained nurses.

It is usually relatively easy to recruit nurses to the DSU because of the sociable hours on duty and its increasingly high profile. However, until recently it was almost impossible to recruit nurses with the necessary qualifications or experience in day surgery (because of the newness of the specialty) and this has resulted in DSUs devising their own training packages for new members of staff. (Training and education is discussed in greater depth in Chapter 9.) On average, it takes at least a year for a nurse to become competent in all aspects of day surgery nursing. This has serious implications in terms of resourcing and skill mix.

Calculating numbers of staff required

It is imperative that the correct establishment for nursing staff is set and maintained. When a new unit is established the number of nurses required is determined by the manager, by taking projected activity levels into consideration. However, when a unit has developed and matured over the years, the nursing staff establishment may never have been adjusted to take into account increasing workload.

To provide safe, effective care, each operating theatre should have a minimum of one anaesthetic assistant and two trained nurses per session. In the first stage recovery area there must be at least one trained nurse per two patients (one for one when caring for children). The ward area should be staffed allowing for one trained nurse per six to eight patients, one nurse for pre-assessment and, ideally, one nurse to take charge of the unit. This information is then converted into hours to give an equation of nursing staff required, as shown in Table 8.1.

Table 8.1: Calculating the number of staff required

Area to be staffed	Nurse hours required	Total
Operating theatre per five hour session	3 x 5 hours	15
Recovery per five hour session	1 x 5 hours	5
		20

The table shows that for one operating session 20 hours of nursing time are needed. This figure is then multiplied by the number of sessions performed per week to give a weekly figure. For example, 20 theatre sessions per week (two operating theatres in use all day, excluding recovery, five days per week) = 300 hours of nursing time. This figure then needs to be broken down into whole time equivalents (WTE), a term used to describe the number of nursing hours available, which may or may not be provided by all full-time staff. The WTE for each nurse is calculated by dividing the number of hours worked by the nurse each week by 37.5 (current full-time hours for nursing staff in the NHS). For example, if a nurse works 23 hours per week, the WTE is 23/37.5, or 0.61 WTE. If two nurses work 23 hours there is a WTE of 1.22, and so on.

So if 300 hours are needed per week to staff the operating theatre safely, dividing this figure by 37.5 gives the number of WTE required (eight) just to staff the two theatres. The hours for the ward area and recovery then need to be added to this figure, and any other activity, such as pre-assessment, minor operations clinics, endoscopy, etc., must also be included into the equation.

Of course, nurses do not work all the time. Each nurse is entitled to five weeks annual leave (under Whitley Council rules) and can be expected to be unwell occasionally. With the implementation of Post-Registration Education and Practice (PREP) there is also a general expectation for time for study (most DSUs are committed to the education of their nurses) and other types of leave. There should, therefore, be an allowance for absence built into the equation. This is known as an uplift and is usually about 20 per cent, which, in the example above, gives a final figure for the operating theatre of 9.6 WTE.

The manager uses these figures when setting the establishment and when arguing for more staff. However, the establishment does not take into account other important factors, such as the skill of the workforce, when staffing a unit. Out of an establishment of 18 WTE there may be 2.5 WTE who are new to day surgery nursing and who require considerable support and training from colleagues. This inevitably puts other nurses under strain and they may perceive the unit as being 'short-staffed' when, in fact, it is up to establishment. Staff may find it difficult to understand why they cannot have additional staff when they feel they are having to work twice as hard as usual. Maternity leave is also often not included in the 20 per cent uplift and this can cause serious staff shortages. Maternity leave should be considered more when it is remembered that a large proportion of the average DSU's staff is female and of child-bearing age.

Perhaps the most important role of the manager is ensuring that there are sufficient nursing staff on duty every day of the week, taking into account all the factors mentioned above. The duty roster or off-duty (as it is more commonly called) has to cover the daily activities of the unit. Such things as level of skill, study leave, requirements of students by the college, individual requests from staff and ensuring that students work with their preceptors (a staff nurse with at least two years' experience in day surgery) at least twice per week all have to be taken into account. There are also legal constraints to be considered, such as the conditions of employment laid down by the Whitley Council, the legal requirement of registered nurses to check controlled drugs and individual contractual agreements about hours worked. Fortunately, it is possible to predict the busiest days in a DSU and the manager soon becomes expert at compiling the roster to ensure there are sufficient members of staff on duty to provide the level of service required at all times.

The use of agency nurses and bank nurses is an option open to managers when trying to cover sickness or absence. However, currently, few, if any, agencies have day surgery trained nurses on their books and may only be able to send either surgical or theatre trained nurses. While they can solve an immediate staffing crisis, this is not the long-term solution to staff shortages and is also expensive for the organisation.

Bank nurses provide a better solution as they can be trained in the DSU itself, are cheaper than agency nurses, are known to the manager and the unit, and will often come into work at very short notice. The nurse manager has a duty not only to the staff of the unit but also to the United Kingdom Central Council for Nursing, Midwifery and Health Visiting (UKCC) to ensure that the unit is adequately covered by nursing staff; failure to do so could constitute an act or omission '… detrimental to the safety of patients' (UKCC, 1984).

Part-time staff are also invaluable to the DSU. As the unit is only open Monday to Friday, many nurses with young children find that the hours of duty suit them well and want to work part-time. The manager is able to fit these hours easily into the working routine because of the regular nature of day surgery. However, there is a risk that too many part-time staff will affect the continuity of care delivered and an almost equal balance of part-time to full-time staff should be attempted. Part-time staff appear to suffer less from high stress levels (Fisher, 1992) and give more when they are at work. However, their full-time colleagues may experience higher stress levels because the onus for maintenance of continuity of care is on them.

The role of non-nursing staff

Operating department practitioners

Although registered nurses form a large proportion of the day surgery team they require considerable help and expertise from other parties. Operating department practitioners (ODPs) are often employed in the DSU, they are qualified personnel who have undergone two years' training at level 3 of the National Vocational Qualification (NVQ) scheme in surgical techniques and anaesthetic care. Because their training is solely within the operating theatre they gain considerable expertise in this field and can contribute greatly to a DSU. They are not qualified to assess or evaluate care in any setting and, therefore, are not able to pre-assess or care for patients in the ward area (other than in a nursing assistant capacity). However, they are often responsible for the maintenance of equipment, day-to-day management and training needs within the theatre suite.

Many hospitals have the policy that only professionals with a qualification in anaesthetic assisting may work with the anaesthetist. Although many nurses are now undertaking ENB 182 (Anaesthetic nursing) or equivalent, there has been a shortage of suitably qualified personnel, and ODPs, because an entire year of their training is taken up with studying anaesthetic care, have traditionally fulfilled this role in many hospitals. Their contribution to the care of the patient in the operating theatre should never be underestimated and they are able to participate in the training of more junior members of staff and those new to day surgery.

However, they are not able to rotate through all the areas of the DSU and are therefore not as flexible as nurses in this particular setting. As the only members of the clinical team who do not participate in all aspects of day surgery care they may feel isolated or even that their role is threatened.

Nursing assistants

This group of unqualified care helpers can also be invaluable to the day surgery team. Many nursing assistants are very experienced in their field and able to provide excellent assistance to the qualified nurse. Nursing assistants are now able to undertake training on the NVQ scheme at either level 2 or 3, which has given them a career structure and improved job satisfaction.

In the DSU, nursing assistants help with the general nursing care of the patient in theatre and ward areas, and prepare refreshments, run errands for patients and staff, assist with clerical duties, 'run' for surgical cases and help to prepare patients for theatre. Their considerable level of contribution to the day surgery team should not underestimated.

Clerical support

No DSU can function successfully without good clerical support. Patient waiting lists need to be administered, appointments arranged, and operating and admissions lists compiled. Since the implementation of the *Patients' Charter* (Department of Health, 1992) a patient must not wait more than one year for surgery and if their surgery is cancelled, for whatever reason, they must receive a new date of admission within a month. Accurate computer records are essential to keep track of patients and to ensure that all are called for surgery when they should be. It falls to clerical assistants, who have received training in the administration of medical records, to keep the records up to date.

Ideally, the DSU admissions office should be sited within the unit itself and have responsibility for controlling all the waiting lists. With this set-up the manager of the DSU is able to monitor the lists and know in advance if specialist equipment is likely to be needed. The non-attendance rate (DNA) of patients is greatly reduced if they are able to have a say in the date of admission and if their date for surgery is not made until they attend for pre-assessment (Solly, 1994). The author suggests that a patient who fails to attend on two separate occasions without explanation has his or her name removed from the waiting list (after a letter has been sent requesting that he or she contact the unit). Patients who do not attend cause considerable inconvenience because an operating slot has been wasted, and in extreme cases extra staff may even have been called in.

In its report on day surgery the NHS Management Executive (1991) recommended that the nurse in charge of the DSU has control over the admissions lists. This results in theatre lists being planned cost-effectively, taking into consideration such elements as the amount of time available and the ability of the surgeon. Therefore, the administration of the DSU waiting lists should be performed separately from the main admissions and waiting lists areas so that the nursing staff have easy access to the admissions office to plan lists and assist patients.

Portering staff

Porters are another essential component of the day surgery team. Although many units use commercial aids for lifting and transferring patients, a porter (or operating department orderly, ODO) is still needed to move patient trolleys, clean the theatre floor between cases, and generally fetch and carry for the staff. Many DSUs, through financial constraint, have to share some, if not all, theatre equipment with the main operating theatres. Therefore, a porter is essential for assisting with the transportation of such equipment between departments.

Ideally, a porter should be employed solely for the DSU. He or she is then able to become familiar not only with the routine of the unit but also with the staff. Being part of the team also fosters a feeling of 'belonging' and loyalty towards the department.

Housekeeping staff

Another vital element of the team is the housekeeping assistant. A DSU, with all its staff and the volume of patients passing through it daily, generates considerable work for housekeeping assistants. Floors need to be washed, toilet areas cleaned and restocked, dusting done and patients' crockery washed up. In many hospitals the domestic staff are also responsible for the thorough daily cleaning of operating theatres. Nurses rarely damp dust and have delegated this responsibility to the housekeeping staff. This group of staff, therefore, have an important role to play within the team. It is the manager's responsibility to ensure that cleanliness standards are maintained. However, it will be the housekeeping staff who will actually implement the standards.

Ideally, all these groups of non-nursing staff should be responsible to the manager of the unit. However, in practice, groups such as porters and housekeeping assistants are often managed separately. This arrangement can work successfully provided the DSU manager retains the authority to dictate requirements.

Team leadership

Every team of people needs a leader as an orchestra needs a conductor (Chapman, 1992). The team leader (manager) must co-ordinate the different levels of expertise and skill within the team. She or he should also ensure that each individual member receives the necessary education and training to fulfil their role. These issues are discussed in greater depth in Chapter 9, but the part the manager plays is briefly examined here.

All nurses new to day surgery should have a preceptor to support and guide them. A structured learning programme helps both the trainee and preceptor. The two should meet and work together regularly. Any problems the trainee is experiencing should be discussed with the manager and strategies planned to help the new nurse gain confidence and achieve competencies. A nurse should not be expected to do anything she or he feels unable to do. Even nurses who come to the unit with previous experience must be allowed to have an orientation period of at least two weeks. This allows them to gain an overview of how the unit works and to familiarise themselves with the routine. It also makes sense for this group to have a 'key worker' – another staff member who has been in post for at least two years – with whom they can discuss difficulties and problems, etc. If these measures are taken when a new staff member is first employed, good morale can be created and maintained by ensuring that everybody has the necessary expertise and confidence for what they are doing. High standards and quality of care are also maintained.

All nurses need education and support, not just those new to day surgery. The manager, in the role as team leader, ensures that all staff are given the opportunity to develop either by attending formal study or by completing a project relevant to their work. New ideas should be discussed and encouraged and support given. Developmental needs are identified at regular appraisal sessions and the manager should aim to appraise every staff member once a year, as well as being available to see staff informally on a regular basis.

Many nurses are worried about the implications of PREP and it is the manager's role to explain these and to guide and help every nurse with her or his own development. Of course, the onus must still lie with the individual nurse to update regularly, but help and guidance must be given and, wherever possible, staff supported, both financially and practically, to attend relevant courses and conferences.

The need for clinical supervision has been realised more in recent years and this role ultimately falls to the most senior nurse (who is often also the manager). Many units now have a specialist nurse for day surgery who has a dual managerial and clinical role and is often paid on the management pay scale. Although this means that standards and professional issues are highlighted, it is a difficult role for the postholder if she or he is still included in the clinical numbers on duty. Ideally, the team leader, whatever the title, should be supernumerary to the clinical team as much as possible to allow time to deal with management and developmental issues. Progressive units should also consider the option of employing a lecturer practitioner jointly with the local faculty of education to provide not only an important link with the university but also to develop training and education both theoretically and clinically.

Higher management structure

So far this chapter has looked only at the management of a DSU at ward level and not at the higher management structure. Each DSU needs to be situated within a well defined management structure.

If a DSU is part of a large general hospital it is important that it creates its own identity and has its own management. If a unit is part of another directorate, for example the anaesthetics and theatre directorate, its needs may not be fully understood in terms of staffing and resources and the DSU may be 'swallowed up' by the requirements of the larger area. Led by the manager, the staff should ensure the unit enjoys a high profile within the hospital by delivering high quality care, an efficient service and becoming a centre of excellence. Ideally, there should also be a clinical director (a consultant with a specialist interest in day surgery) who is able to work alongside the manager and positively promote the work of the DSU.

Clinical directorates

A clinical director is able to support the DSU and represent it at Board level. He or she is likely to be respected by other colleagues for his or her clinical competence as well as managerial skills and therefore carries some credence when difficult or controversial issues have to be debated. The clinical director has several roles: negotiator, financial manager, contracts manager, conciliator and organiser, although some of these components may be delegated to a specialty general manager.

As day surgery develops, it is essential for each unit to have an effective director to take this growth forward. A doctor provides a stable influence within hospital management, which often changes completely every few years. However, the clinical director is not able to override other medical colleagues' professional judgement and individual consultants must retain continuing responsibility for their patients. Not all senior doctors possess the attributes required to be a successful manager; many prefer to remain solely in the clinical field and some are suspicious of management.

The clinical directorate structure was established in the early 1990s. It has led to more focused management and a clearer sense of direction for those who provide health care (Nichol & Turnberg, 1993). A clinical directorate is a clinical specialty made up of several consultants. It is led by a consultant clinician and the directorate takes responsibility for its own budget and affairs, including nursing and paramedical staff.

It is debatable in which directorate a DSU should be placed. Day surgery provides a support service to the other surgical directorates in that it supplies a day surgery facility. When the DSU is part of another surgical management structure, its special needs may either be ignored or a biased approach unwittingly taken. A good solution is to place it in the operational services directorate.

Different designs of day surgical unit

Everybody involved in the provision of day surgery care will have their own views as to what constitutes the 'ideal DSU'. This section examines the advantages and disadvantages of each model, and the author gives her opinion on each.

There are three main ways in which day surgery care may be delivered:

- in a self-contained unit within a hospital;
- in a self-contained unit separate from a hospital;
- in a day surgery ward making use of main theatre time.

It is also worth mentioning that in some hospitals, day surgical patients are cared for in a general surgical ward and the problems associated with the management of these patients are also considered.

Self-contained unit within a hospital

A self-contained unit can be defined as a ward area catering for patients pre- and post-operatively and an operating theatre (or suite) solely for day patients situated within the same area. Both areas are staffed by day surgery staff and are managed by one manager. In their research, Jones et al. (1992) compared the throughput of patients in their dedicated DSU with that of the main theatre block. They found that the speed with which patients were 'delivered' to theatre was three to four times quicker in the DSU than in the main theatre. They therefore conclude that a dedicated, self-contained unit is essential for maximum efficiency.

The advantages of this set-up are that all the staff are trained and proficient in the specialist care required by those undergoing day surgery. Beds cannot be used for emergency admissions and the unit is designed to facilitate the easy passage of patients. It is relatively easy to manage, as all the staff are working in the same area and managerial, clinical support services and emergency support are all available from the rest of the hospital.

Some units have been designed to the 'race track' specification (see Figure 8.1). This, broadly speaking, means that the patient moves through a pre-operative area, anaesthetics, surgery and, finally, to the post-operative area in circular motion. Consequently, pre- and post-operative patients are not mixed.

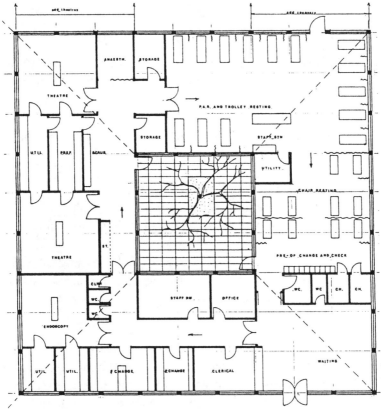

Figure 8.1: Race track design of day surgical unit
Previously published in the Journal of One Day Surgery and reproduced with the permission of the publishers, Newton Mann Ltd.

Disadvantages are that this style of unit can cause difficulties in staffing as the pre- and post-operative sections are separate. Patients may gain the impression that they are on a conveyor belt. The author can see no necessity for separating pre- and post-operative patients and has found that post-operative patients can help to reduce pre-operative anxiety, as patients waiting for surgery are pleasantly surprised by the fitness of those who have already had surgery.

Units situated within a hospital have the benefit of support from the rest of the organisation, e.g. X-ray, pathology and central sterile supplies (CSSD). In the event of a critical incident help is quickly at hand. However, as mentioned in the previous section, the unit may be 'swallowed up' by the rest of the hospital and its staff not given the recognition they deserve for their expertise and knowledge. Day surgery nursing is often perceived by other nurses as a soft option because the hours are usually sociable and there is not much 'hands on', traditional nursing to be done. As only relatively minor surgery is carried out, patients are normally fit, and the DSU may be seen as the least important service of the hospital with the lowest priority patients. It may be the first area to be closed in times of strife when funding is low. Day surgery may not have the glamour of the high powered services of intensive therapy or transplant surgery, but to its patients it is just as important and in some instances, life-saving.

'Stand-alone' day surgical units

This type of DSU is on a different site from a hospital. It may be entirely separate both physically and managerially or may still be administered by the hospital to which it is affiliated.

In the USA, DSUs are often situated separately from a hospital and there are some such 'stand-alone' units in this country. They may be sited several miles away from the nearest hospital and many professionals fear this system because of the lack of emergency help when required.

Some stand-alone units have been established in old hospitals that have been rendered redundant by changes in health care but still retain out-patient and other services. And in some places general practitioners have set up day surgery services attached to their surgeries. As long as the potential problems are considered from the outset there is no reason why this type of unit cannot be as successful, if not more so, than its counterpart at the general hospital. The unit is not subject to hospital interference in terms of political moves (Powell, 1995) and is able to run along the lines the staff themselves wish and not those that may be imposed from on high.

However, there are inevitable difficulties that can arise when a unit is apart from a hospital. For example, a patient who needs to be admitted for an overnight stay will have to be taken there by ambulance, which can cause delays and inconvenience to both patient and staff. This can largely be avoided by careful, accurate pre-assessment of all patients and by placing patients considered at risk of needing an overnight bed at the beginning of the list, so allowing more time for recovery and to arrange an ambulance if necessary.

An emergency situation can arise at any time and cannot be predicted. It is, therefore, vital that all staff are regularly updated in their resuscitation skills, that only senior medical staff attend day surgery patients and that well maintained, state-of-the-art emergency equipment is available at all times. The anaesthetist should not leave the unit until the nurse in charge is happy that all patients have recovered sufficiently from anaesthesia, and nurses must always know how and where to contact the anaesthetist and surgeon should they need to do so. The number of nurses on duty must also reflect the fact that in an emergency they may be on their own for some time and there must be a sufficient number to enable them to deal with the situation and to summon help.

Despite the concerns outlined above, the author considers stand-alone units to be the best option and believes that the day surgery/treatment centre will become increasingly common. These could be run by consortia of hospital consultants, GPs and community trusts.

Shared facilities

Providing day surgery care through the sharing of facilities is probably the least favourable option. The most common arrangement is that a ward is set aside for day surgery patients and their surgery is performed in the main theatre.

Day patients have totally different needs from in-patients. The speed of care required means that the use of main theatre time is usually unsatisfactory. Main theatre staff will not be used to the high turnover of patients or be as skilled in delivering the high quality care required by day patients. Junior medical staff may be employed to administer anaesthetics, which is not recommended (Royal College of Surgeons, 1992), and the theatre may be situated some distance from the ward where post-operative care is delivered. When day patients are 'slotted in' between more major cases and left for the junior surgeon to operate on, the status of the day surgery patient is reduced and, therefore, quality of care is compromised. If there is no alternative but to use an operating theatre within the main suite, one theatre should be set aside for the use of the day surgery unit so that it can be equipped and staffed with day patients in mind. Ideally, the day theatre staff should be managed by the DSU to ensure the maintenance of standards of care.

There are many problems associated with this way of delivering care and, in the author's opinion, this method should only be employed if there is absolutely no other option. However, it is preferable to caring for day patients within a general ward. In this setting, day patients may not receive the psychological care and the meticulous preparation they require. Day patients may be perceived as a low priority compared with the other, sicker patients nursed in the ward. They often have to wait for a bed to become available, have only a superficial assessment and scant attention is paid to their needs. Little, if any, post-operative advice or information is given and vital instructions may be omitted. This is not the fault of the nursing or medical staff of these wards, they simply have not received the specialist training required for caring for day surgery patients and do not physically have the time to devote to them. A busy surgical ward is certainly not the place for the day surgery patient.

Designing a new day surgical unit

Some hospitals are fortunate enough to have a DSU built to their specifications and there has been much written about the way a unit should be designed. Other hospitals have to adapt existing buildings with limited finance and are not necessarily able to have the unit to the specifications they would have chosen. However, it is possible to design an efficient unit whichever approach is taken.

Before designing a unit a committee should be established. This should consist of the estates manager for the hospital, a consultant surgeon or anaesthetist, an architect, a senior nurse and the project administrator. This group should consider the number of patients to be treated, the types of surgery to be performed and the way in which care will be managed. It is generally considered practical to site a DSU on the ground floor close to ample car parking, with its own entrance separate to that of the hospital. It makes sense to situate the DSU close to the out-patient department and to the CSSD, if possible. This facilitates ease of movement for the patient and easy transfer of sterile supplies.

A pleasant environment should be created to minimise the 'institutional' feel so often associated with older hospitals. The DSU should have the qualities of a first-class hotel, and a well designed interior can reduce anxiety and stress and inspire confidence in the level of service provided (McTaggart, 1993).

A self-contained DSU should have sufficient bed space for the number of patients to be treated and an appropriate number of operating theatres with associated anaesthetic rooms, store cupboards and recovery area. There has been some debate on whether or not anaesthetic rooms are necessary in DSUs. Most anaesthetists tend to induce anaesthesia in the operating theatre as this saves time and reduces the need for moving anaesthetised patients. However, the decision to exclude anaesthetic rooms should be considered carefully. Anaesthetic rooms are useful when treating children and for use as a minor treatment room while the operating theatre is in use. They are also used for the storage of essential equipment that needs to be kept close to the operating theatre.

There should be sufficient office space for both management and medical staff. If the admission of patients is to be administered from within the unit, offices and storage areas for patient files must also be created. Waiting rooms should be pleasantly designed and comfortable, and there should be adequate toilet facilities for both patients and staff. Areas for making refreshments for patients must be provided, and there should be comfortable and practical staff rest areas, with sufficient changing areas.

Everyone has their own ideas on the ideal design of a DSU. All these views should be taken into consideration when redesigning an existing building or erecting a new one. Broadly speaking, the building should reflect the philosophy of the unit by being user-friendly, comfortable and non-institutional, while at the same time being functional, efficient and cost-effective. Some parties favour the 'race-track' design where a patient moves around the unit through the different stages of treatment. Others prefer a definite distinction between ward areas and operating theatres as this is easier to staff. Whichever design is chosen, it is the quality of care delivered which ultimately matters and this must be of a high level whatever the environment.

Recent NHS reforms and their effect on day surgery

The recent changes in the organisation of the NHS are worthy of mention in relation to the growth of day surgery in the UK. There will no doubt be future changes which will affect the ways in which care is delivered.

The effect of the White Paper

The aim of the changes to the NHS, which were announced in the White Paper *Working for Patients* (Department of Health, 1989) was to improve the performance and service offered by all hospitals and GPs. Previously, funding of the health service in the UK had been 'buildings-led' (Teasdale, 1992, p. 2). The larger inner city hospitals received more funding regardless of the demography of the area. This resulted in some out of town areas receiving less funding than a large inner city hospital. The provincial hospital may have considerable demands on its services, particularly if a large proportion of the population it serves are elderly. This group of patients may also have moved out of the inner city area.

The ideologies of the White Paper were that a funding system be introduced that uses census figures to monitor population trends. Public money is, therefore, divided in such a way as to reflect the changes in the population. The principle is that money follows the patient, and GPs have greater freedom over where to send their patients for treatment. This in turn, creates an atmosphere of competition. A hospital that can attract a larger number of patients can increase its income.

An internal market of purchasers and providers was created. The purchasers have the responsibility of using public money to buy health services on behalf of patients. The purchaser is usually the District Health Authority (DHA) and its role is to assess the needs of the population it serves and to buy health care from any provider that offers good service and value for money.

These changes resulted in providers having greater freedom in the way in which their units are run. Day surgery is generally believed to be a cost-effective method of providing surgery for more minor conditions. Cost savings from day surgery have been widely reported (Bailey, 1993; Bridger & Rees, 1995; Fawcett-Henesy, 1995). However, these cost savings have to be set against the high cost of establishing a DSU. A DSU also stands idle at weekends and this has to be offset by the intensity of use during the working week.

It is clear that day surgery has expanded out of a desire for achieving financial savings and value for money. It is debatable whether this development would have occurred at the pace of the last few years without the implementation of the White Paper.

The role of the GP

Since the NHS reforms, the GP's role has, in some instances, been altered. Larger GP practices have been able to become holders of public money in the same way as DHAs. They are known as GP fundholders. They are able to dictate the quality and type of treatment that their patients receive and negotiate over price because they control some of the funds needed by the provider to run their services. This could result in patients from fundholding practices receiving quicker or better treatment from hospitals that are anxious to win contracts in order to secure finance. It may also mean that GPs make fewer referrals in the interests of cost reduction. Day surgery, in particular, could suffer as a result of this as more GP practices establish minor surgery clinics within their own premises.

GP practices that are not large enough or do not wish to be fundholding remain the providers of services to the patient. They still retain the freedom to refer their patients to whomever they wish, theoretically, anywhere in the country. However, most have agreed to remain with the previous referral pattern of using local providers.

It has become imperative for DSUs to attract patients from fundholding GPs. The impact of public opinion on purchasers, especially fundholders (Edmondson & Billings, 1995), must also be considered. The quality of service must, therefore, be high. This issue is examined later in the chapter.

NHS trusts

Many hospital units have acquired so called 'trust status' in recent years. This means that the hospital (or community care unit) controls its own affairs. It is responsible for securing money from the purchasers and cannot automatically turn to the DHA if it runs into difficulty. Trusts have the freedom to decide how to manage capital assets, such as buildings, land or equipment, and can also make decisions on terms and conditions for staff. They are reliant on the purchaser for funding and can negotiate contracts for the provision of health care.

However, the purchaser is also able to buy health care from the independent sector if it so chooses. This has the effect of some NHS trusts being in direct competition with private hospitals for some aspects of health care. Therefore, contracts for certain services are vital to determine the amount of money that the provider will receive.

It must be remembered, however, that the success of the DSU in terms of financial support is dependent on the quality of service offered. As already mentioned, GPs and DHAs have far greater say in the quality and speed of treatment they purchase. The *Patients' Charter* (Department of Health, 1992) dictates how long a patient has to wait for surgery and the waiting list times also influence the awarding of contracts by the purchaser.

Audit

It is clear from the previous section that in order to survive, providers of health care must secure contracts. Part of this process is the delivery of good service and care. Patients who believe their care to be below standard will quickly report this to their GP. If the GP happens to be a fundholder, a contract may not be renewed. Similarly, a contract may be awarded to an alternative provider who is able to offer better service at a lower price.

Measuring and monitoring service and care

Over the past 20 years or so there has been a gradual shift of opinion as to the levels of service that can be expected from the public sectors. The population now has an expectation of receiving the same standards of care and service as that previously found only in the private sector of health care. These changes are largely due to government initiatives such as the *Patients' Charter* (1992) and, although generally favourably received by health care professionals, have had the effect of increasing their workload.

Standards

'Quality' became a nursing buzzword during the 1980s and has now been more or less totally embraced by the profession as an essential component of good practice. By measuring the standard of care and service provided, change may be introduced, which may then be monitored and changed again if indicated. This may be seen by some as change for change sake. In fact, when audit is implemented properly and enthusiastically it has the effect of fostering not only high standards but also good morale among staff. A stimulating and happy atmosphere is created for the benefit of both patients and staff. To ascertain whether or not something is effective it has to be measured against a standard. If you go into a shop and ask for a kilogram of potatoes you are happy in the knowledge that you will receive a certain amount of potatoes because a kilogram is a standard weight that is recognised internationally. If you are given less than a kilogram you are able to complain in the knowledge that you did not receive exactly the amount you asked for.

This same principle may be applied when setting standards in the workplace. The first step is to decide what aspect of care or service needs to have a standard. Once that has been agreed a process of 'structure, process, outcome' is implemented. This framework was first described by Donabedian (1969) and has been widely adopted by the nursing profession. There are various other methods for the setting of standards and audit packs are available commercially.

The audit cycle

A process for measuring outcomes against the standard has to be implemented. 'Audit' literally means examination and that is exactly what is happening when the audit cycle is set in progress. The service or care is being examined.

For audit to be successful, three components are required – time, tools and training. Time is needed for all parties to understand the audit cycle, agree the priorities, agree methods, actually carry out the audit, collate and consider the results, and implement change in response to findings. For the data to be collected a format needs to be devised that is repeatable and simple. All parties concerned with the audit process need to be trained in its use and how the findings might affect them. It is natural for people to feel threatened by audit. They may feel they are being watched or criticised and may not understand why change is necessary, especially when a procedure has been in place for many years with no apparent problems. The question the manager should pose to those who doubt the usefulness of audit is 'How do we know that this method works?'.

There are several audit packages available on the market that have been devised specifically for nursing projects and these may be easily adapted for use in the DSU. It is recommended that before the manager instigates a new method of audit in the workplace, she or he receives training in the audit process. The manager should be well conversant in the differing methods, have widely read around the subject and have the ability to infuse the staff involved with enthusiasm for audit. Some examples of possible audit subjects in the DSU are given in Table 8.2, all of which have probably been audited by various DSUs in the UK.

Table 8.2: Possible audit subjects in the DSU

Non-clinical	*Clinical*
Length of waiting lists	Rate of post-operative admission for overnight stays
Patient satisfaction with service	Incidence of post-operative nausea and vomiting
Efficacy of written information leaflets	Pain after surgery

Before embarking on an audit, a literature search should be performed. This helps to give ideas for the preferred method of audit, expected outcomes and prevents repetition. Approval must also be sought and obtained from the Ethics Committee for the trust or organisation. Ethics committees are set up by the medical profession to vet research projects. Their purpose is to protect the potential subject of research and they are sensitive to the need for confidentiality (Cormack, 1991). The findings should then be published. If the results are particularly interesting, national publication might be considered. Quality of care improves if knowledge and research findings are shared.

There are many texts available on the subject of audit and further reading is advisable before implementation of an audit in the workplace.

The audit cycle and staff

The implementation of a formal process of audit in the DSU can have the effect of significantly increasing the workload on the nursing and medical staff. This in turn can cause resentment among staff who may already feel that they are being asked to perform the impossible by management. Devolving 'ownership' of audit down to the staff helps to overcome these feelings. Staff feel that they are involved and are a critical component to improving and maintaining high standards. All nurses want to provide the best care possible for their patients and once the important role of audit in monitoring these high standards is explained, will become enthusiastic about the audit cycle. It is, therefore, crucial that all staff are included when an audit cycle is planned. Not all may want to be directly involved in the actual collection and collation of data, but all will want to know the outcomes and how their practice can be improved.

Some DSUs are fortunate enough to be able to employ a nurse whose sole job is to undertake audit and some NHS trusts employ an audit nurse on whose services the DSU may call. Where these personnel are available they should be used effectively. Day surgery nurses have a difficult task in performing the best for their patients, and audit is frequently seen as an unnecessary, time-consuming chore.

The DSU managers must present audit as a positive process that enhances nursing and medical care of the patient. The entire team should be actively involved in the process and the individual members encouraged to view audit as an exciting challenge, which they are keen to meet.

Summary

The role of the manager in the DSU is multifaceted and orchestrates the workings of the unit. It is a role that should not be undertaken lightly and without training and experience in the specialty. The manager will often face criticism from staff, medical colleagues and higher management and will have to deal with difficult situations involving personal feelings.

The first priority of the manager must always be the safe and effective care of the patients passing through the unit and she or he must also ensure that there is compliance with local and national policy at all times. A good manager is one who can juggle all the differing components but still retain a sense of humour, empathy, compassion and, perhaps most important of all, clinical credence. In these days of cost cutting and financial awareness the manager will often have to impose unpopular measures to ensure efficiency and economy, but by maintaining good communication channels and listening to the views of staff and patients she or he can ensure a smooth-running, efficient and happy DSU.

It is hoped that this chapter will help all aspiring DSU managers to achieve these goals and encourage further reading and study on the subject.

References

Bailey JM (1993) Day surgery: a problem of economics or financial management? Ambulatory Surgery 1(3): 125–128.

Bridger P, Rees M (1995) What a difference a day makes. Health Service Journal 105(5449): 22–23.

Chapman G (1992) What is management? In Horne E, Cowan T (Eds), Ward Sister's Survival Guide. London: Wolfe Publishing.

Cormack DSF (1991) The Research Process in Nursing, 2nd edn. Oxford: Blackwell Scientific Publications.

Department of Health (1989) Working for Patients. London: HMSO.

Department of Health (1992) The Patients' Charter. London: HMSO.

Donabedian A (1969) Evaluating the quality of medical care. Millbank Memorial Fund Quarterly 4: 166–203.

Edmondson M, Billings J (1995) G.P. Fundholders: marketing day surgery – a personal view. Surgical Nurse 8(2): 29–31.

Fawcett-Henesy A (1995) All right on the day? Nursing Standard 9(43): 52.

Fisher J (1992) Part-time staff: a blessing in disguise? In Horne M, Cowan T (Eds), Ward Sister's Survival Guide. London: Wolfe Publishing.

Jones A, Greaves K, Parker C, Briggs T, Miller R (1992) The case for a day case unit. Journal of One Day Surgery 2(2): 11–14.

McTaggart R (1993) Policies for the planning of day surgery units. Journal of One Day Surgery 2(4): 10–11.

NHS Management Executive (1991) Day Surgery – Making it Happen. London: HMSO.

Nichol D, Turnberg L (1993) Foreword. In Hopkins A (Ed), The Role of the Hospital Consultant in Clinical Directorates. London: Royal College of Physicians.

Powell J (1995) All on our own: away from the District Hospital. Journal of One Day Surgery 5(2): 11.

Royal College of Surgeons (1992) Report of the Working Party on Guidelines for Day Case Surgery. London: RCS.

Solly J (1994) Tackling do not attend rates in day surgery. Journal of One Day Surgery 4(2): 28–29.

Sutherland R (1994) Is this the way forward? British Journal of Theatre Nursing 4(1): 12–13.

Teasdale K (1992) Managing the Changes in Health Care. London: Wolfe.

United Kingdom Central Council for Nursing, Midwifery and Health Visiting (1984) Code of Professional Conduct for the Nurse, Midwife and Health Visitor. London: UKCC.

Further reading

Gilchrist B (1992) Writing the off-duty. In Horne M, Cowan T (Eds), Ward Sister's Survival Guide. London: Wolfe Publishing.

Gould T, Merrett H (1992) Introducing Quality Assurance into the NHS. Basingstoke: The MacMillan Press.

Hopkins A (Ed) (1993) The Role of Hospital Consultants in Clinical Directorates – The Synchromesh Report. London: Royal College of Physicians.

White T (1994) Management for Clinicians. London: Edward Arnold.

Chapter 9
Education and training for day surgery nurses

Debbie Green

Introduction

Whether you have read through this book in detail or just skimmed the chapter titles, you will by now be aware that the role of the day surgery nurse is multifaceted, providing pre- and post-operative care, anaesthetic care, surgical care and recovery care for all age-groups. The choice of the word 'multifaceted' is intentional. Many managers appear to prefer the word 'multiskilled'. Definitions of this latter word pale into insignificance compared with the debate either for or against the concept. Reid (1995) reported on the 1995 Royal College of Nurses Congress, where some speakers saw multiskilling for trained nurses as a threat, with untrained personnel replacing them because they were cheaper. Proponents of multiskilling state that nursing staff 'will acquire a great range of skills and be able to contribute in a more flexible approach to patient-centred care' (Kenworthy, 1995, p. 33).

Links have been made between multiskilling and the day surgery setting in recent years. Like the concept itself, this is a controversial issue; some authors, including Penn (1990), support it and others, including Sutherland (1994), question whether multiskilling is appropriate in the day surgery setting. However, there is no doubt that day surgery nurses have to be flexible and adaptable to cope with the increasing range of surgical and medical specialties and the fast throughput of patients.

The controversy surrounding multiskilling will undoubtly continue, and rightly so. Perhaps the message to portray is that the concept requires discussion at a local level and within individual day surgical units (DSUs), as it can be influenced by a number of conditions, including the number, grades and competency of staff (nursing and non-nursing), the number of operating theatres and associated anaesthetic and surgical procedures, and the additional services provided for patient care, such as endoscopy and laser therapy.

Whether you consider day surgery nurses to be multiskilled or their role to be multifaceted, they require education and training. This chapter will explore why education and training for all staff are important. It will consider professional courses for trained nurses and share some ideas for the clinical placement of diploma students. In addition, it will examine clinical updating for staff, notably the recent professional developments and 'in-house' learning, and consider the future of day surgery education.

Why are education and training important?

Staff working within a DSU are undertaking work that only a decade ago took place in a number of settings – the ward, theatre, recovery and back to the ward. Whatever the setting, technology has also made an impact on patient care, but particularly within the theatre environment where staff are having to come to terms with new pharmacology, laryngeal masks, minimal access techniques and laser procedures. Additionally, surgical procedures in DSUs have progressed from minor cases (such as removal of lipomas, sebaceous cysts and ingrowing toe-nails) to intermediate cases (such as tonsillectomy, laparoscopic cholecystectomy and retinal detatchment). Some trusts have purposefully called their units 'day treatment centres', which enables medical procedures like blood transfusions and cytotoxic therapies to be given to patients.

But do all staff have the necessary specific competencies for every specialty? Before attempting to answer this, it may be more appropriate to consider some of the generic knowledge and competencies required. This kind of education and training is particularly important for new staff being oriented to a unit and it covers areas such as health and safety, risk management and, for nurses, professional issues.

The Health and Safety at Work Act 1974 requires employers to provide an environment for employees that is healthy and safe. For staff working in a day surgery unit, this includes aspects of care such as moving and handling, spillages, fire regulations and documentation. In units that do not have operating trolleys for patients, unconscious patients have to be transferred manually from operating table to trolley, and then possibly from trolley to bed. Whichever staff member carries out these procedures, they must conform to the minimum safety requirements for manual handling operations initiated by the European Community in 1990 and brought into force on 1 January 1993. This means they should be able to undertake a risk assessment, know how to transfer patients correctly, theoretically and practically, and the appropriate aids should be available to prevent back injury, with the staff member knowing how to access the aid and how to use it appropriately. The responsibility for this training rests with the employer, as does the provision of aids. However, the DSU manager also has a responsibility to ensure that staff are released for such training as is provided. The onus is on the individual practitioner, too, to have a good knowledge of recent legislation so they can start to agitate if they do not feel adequate education, training or resources are in place.

A DSU contains potentially dangerous materials and equipment, for example, volatile anaesthetic agents, surgical diathermy, lasers and oxygen. These items are capable of contributing to fire. Staff members need to know the telephone number to call to raise the alarm. They need to be aware of the differences in alarm sounds (the meaning of intermittent and continuous rings, depending on the hospital protocol). Staff need to know the appropriate extinguishing apparatus for the type of fire, where these apparatus are kept in the DSU and how to use them. They should also know the location of fire exits and how to evacuate patients, carers and staff through them. It all sounds straightforward, but questioning staff – old and new – about some of the points above is likely to produce some surprising answers.

Spillages are a further concern. Patients who attend a DSU are likely to have an invasive procedure, thus staff could come into contact with blood and body fluids which have the potential to harbour hepatitus B virus or human immunodeficiency virus. Universal Precautions have been advocated for over 20 years by the Center for Disease Control in Atlanta, USA, yet some staff still look amazed if their practices are challenged. Universal Precautions advocate that all patients should be cared for in the same manner because health care staff have no idea which patients have contracted communicable diseases. Universal Precautions also protect health care staff through the use of protective clothing and eyewear, and minimal handling of sharps (Taylor, 1993). Staff who would like more information regarding Universal Precautions are advised to contact their occupational health department.

A brief mention should be made of more recent health and safety legislation, the Control of Substances Hazardous to Health

(COSHH). These regulations came into force late in 1989. They have far reaching consequences in all health care settings, but perhaps the one most relevant in the DSU is the use of glutaraldehyde. This solution is currently the most effective disinfectant for use on equipment that cannot be autoclaved (for example, rigid and fibre-optic endoscopes). However, care must be taken when using it. It is highly irritant to the skin and the membranes lining the gastric and respiratory systems, therefore, staff must be aware of the precautions needed to protect themselves and the patient. Staff must wear gloves and protective clothing and eyewear, and the use of special enclosed washing machines in well ventilated areas is advocated. As with all equipment, staff must be trained to use it properly, and the manufacturer of the washing machine should offer not only a maintenance programme but also a teaching package for users. Staff can be further trained via a cascade system whereby staff trained by the manufacturer's representative train staff who were unable to attend the official training session. Parties with a particular interest in endoscopy can take ENB 906 (Care of patients undergoing gastrointestinal endoscopy and related procedures) to expand their theory and practice in this area.

A good source of more detailed information on COSHH are the reports published by the British Society of Gastroenterologists.

Documentation is now essential in health care. Kalideen (1991) listed five reasons for recording information – evidence for continuous care; evidence for quality care; improved communication; evidence of evaluation; and information for litigation. In 1993 the United Kingdom Central Council (UKCC) produced a leaflet for nursing staff offering guidance on record-keeping, stressing that it is an integral part of nursing. In the day surgery setting, most units are now adopting multidisciplinary notes, where the medical staff in the out-patients department document the initial patient details. These notes then follow the patient through pre-assessment and admission on the day of surgery, the documentation being completed by a registered nurse. The surgeon and anaesthetist have the opportunity to complete their respective sections for the operative phase. These notes are concluded by the registered nurse who discharges the patient and carer home. Where there is a supporting role between a DSU and community services, for example, a Hospital at Home scheme, multidisciplinary notes have an extra section for the documentation of such continuing care provision.

The advantage of multidisciplinary notes is that they become the point of reference for all health care professionals who come into contact with the patient. In addition to the staff already mentioned, these may include a physiotherapist following a patient undergoing an arthroscopy or a family planning nurse following a patient who has just had a termination of pregnancy. The disadvantages of multi-disciplinary notes are that they can become rather large and unwieldy – up to 20 pages in some instances. They can also be repetitive if they are not carefully constructed and this is aggravating for patients and time-consuming for staff.

Risk management has become necessary in the health service for two principal reasons – the loss of Crown immunity and the financial responsibilities of trust hospitals. Roy (1996) says risk management can be described as the opportune identification and management of existing risk, to facilitate the protection of all parties concerned. Any risk management strategies should be considered on an individual ward or department basis, as risks will be peculiar to that individual area. This is particularly relevant to day surgery as DSUs are often separate or distant from other facilities to which they have links, for example, out-patients and main theatres.

Risk management in the health service is concerned with both non-clinical and clinical issues. The former often relate to failure to comply with health and safety regulations, which has already been touched upon, and the latter relates to care and treatment in the DSU. Care and treatment issues include patient selection and pre-assessment; surgical procedures; patient recovery and discharge; and DSU personnel (Hill & Roberts, 1992). Using the last point to illustrate the Roy (1996) description means personnel should be experienced and able to cope competently with any emergency that may arise, whether they are medical or nursing staff, operating department personnel (ODP) or clerical staff. This last group can be taught basic first aid, which can increase their skills repetoire, make them feel more integrated into the team and ultimately enhance patient care.

Professional issues for nursing staff must relate to the Code of Professional Practice (UKCC, 1992a) and the Scope of Professional Practice (UKCC, 1992b). There are three clauses of the Code that deal specifically with education.

Clause 3: 'maintain and improve your professional knowledge and competence'. Day surgery is a young and growing specialty. For nurses working in this area it is essential to keep abreast of numerous issues, for example: new nursing developments, such as post-operative telephone follow-ups or information sheets for carers to clarify their responsibilities; and new anaesthetic and surgical techniques, such as the quest for more effective analgesics and anti-emetics, and the increasing number of operations that can be performed as minimally invasive techniques. Challenging links between the primary and acute sectors will no doubt occur as more intermediate procedures are undertaken. Much has been written about having a community-based nurse attached to the DSU and perhaps this will become commonplace as we move toward the next millenium.

Keeping up to date can be achieved by talking to colleagues working in the same field, which is why the British Association of Day Surgery (BADS) Annual Conference is so popular. Nurses can telephone or visit other local DSUs to ask for information, or see how they function. Books and journals are a further source of information and these are often listed at the back of Audit Commission and National Health Service Management Executive Reports on day surgery. A computerised literature search will produce extra material on your given topic as so many journals now have articles related to day surgery – paediatric; care of the elderly; intensive care.

The concept of competence is itself controversial. The ENB (1990a) definition is 'the ability to perform a particular activity to a prescribed standard', but this sounds rather task-oriented and may be interpreted in that manner by managers. The definition offered by Gale and Pol (1977), although dated, has a more encompassing view: competence is 'the abilities, skills, judgement, attitudes and values required for successful functioning'. This is surely how we would wish day surgery nurses to be considered in terms of their competence. There is also the issue of who should decide nursing competence. One viewpoint is that day surgery nursing competence should be debated nationally (for example, at the BADS conference) to enable a framework to be constructed. This framework could then be adapted for use at a local level. Contributors to the debate should include managers, practitioners and educationalists. If such a framework could be constructed it would allow nurses to move geographically (for whatever reason), recording their competence via the post-registration education and practice (PREP) documentation and presenting it to their new or prospective employer. This would provide the manager with a complete insight into the nurse's achievements and competence during her or his previous employment.

Clause 4: 'acknowledge any limitations in your knowledge and competence and decline any duties or responsibilities unless able to perform them in a safe and skilled manner'. With the short amount of time patients now spend in hospital, it is vital that patients receive the correct care and information to safeguard them when they return to their own homes. Failure to do so will place them at considerable risk. If a nurse fails to inform the patient of the importance of not operating machinery for the first 24 hours, and the patient decides to do some cooking while still affected by their general anaesthetic and sustains a burn, then the nurse is negligent. This therefore means that only nurses who have been trained to discharge a patient should do so. Nurses new to the day surgery setting should be adequately supervised before being given such a role.

In the present climate of cost restraint and increasing work pressures, a nurse may be tempted to perform a role for which she or he has not been adequately trained, misguidedly thinking she or he is acting in the best interests of the patient, but the consequences of this can be dire. Once patients have been discharged from the DSU they can only contact the health care professionals if they have problems, because staff do not have time to contact every patient on a routine basis. In-patients' problems can be monitored in hospital and advice given on an ongoing basis. This is a luxury not afforded to day surgery patients. Poorly prepared staff who have the potential to make mistakes (because they do not acknowledge knowledge or practice gaps) will only hinder rather than enhance day surgery patient care. This may ultimately lead to bad publicity or the loss of general practitioner (GP) contracts.

Clause 14: 'assist professional colleagues, in the context of your own knowledge, experience and sphere of responsibility, to develop their professional competence, and assist others in the care team, including informal carers, to contribute safely and to a degree appropriate to their roles'. BADS promotes day surgery as a multidisciplinary specialty so it has recognised the importance of information sharing. However, does this occur in reality?

Our medical colleagues appear to have the upper hand if the number of articles contributed to the two leading day surgery journals - the British *Journal of One Day Surgery* and the international *Ambulatory Surgery* journal, are anything to go by. But if we turn this scenario on its head then maybe we are not giving nurses the necessary support and encouragement to publish. If this support was available then nurses may acquire the confidence to argue their views personally in the literature and publically in users' committees for their own DSU or, on a larger scale, at national or international conferences.

In relation to the assistance for carers, it could be argued that day surgery would not be the success it is but for the large (and growing) role of carers. Carers are having to perform the previously traditional role of the surgical ward nurse. Their responsibilities include encouraging the patient to rest/mobilise in adequate amounts; provision of refreshments; observation of complications such as swelling and/or pain; and contacting the appropriate persons if help should be required (Green, 1995).

Information relating to their role should be shared with the carer if they attend the pre-assessment interview with the patient. This should be reinforced when the carer returns to collect the patient on the day of surgery. There can be problems if the carer cannot attend the pre-assessment, or if the escort taking the patient home is a different person from the carer. The patient should be given written information that they can share with their families/neighbours and that will act as an aide-mémoire for themselves.

Chapter 2 has shown that pre-assessment is an essential phase of care for the day surgery patient. The skills needed for pre-assessment are best discussed using Bloom's (1956) taxonomy – cognitive, psychomotor and affective. In the cognitive domain, the nurse should be sound in her or his knowledge and understanding of the medical and social criteria for day surgery. Additionally, as a patient educator, the day surgery nurse should have a thorough knowledge of anaesthetic and surgical procedures, and the necessary after-care. The psychomotor domain requires the nurse to have excellent communication skills, particularly listening skills, questioning skills and the identification and analysis of patient cues. The ability to form relationships and exchange information relates to the nurse's interpersonal behaviours and probably best falls into the affective domain. Finally, the nurse requires good record-keeping skills, with the capacity to write clearly and concisely on the patient's multidisciplinary notes. These categories could be used for principal competency areas to be achieved under supervision with a more experienced colleague in the learning situation.

The Scope of Professional Practice (UKCC, 1992b) was designed to overcome the extended role, which tended to be based on particular activities and not on the holistic nursing role. The principles for adjusting the Scope of Practice and how these can be applied in the day surgery setting are discussed below.

1.   *'must be satisfied that each aspect of practice is directed to meeting the needs and serving the interests of the patient or client'*. What are the needs of the day surgery patient? The *Day Surgery Task Force Report* (NHSME, 1993a) gives the consumers' needs as firstly, the provision of adequate and relevant information (oral and

written) at the appropriate time along the patient's 'journey'. Secondly, the provision of help and support from health care staff at hospital and when they return home. To this end, many DSUs now have a mobile telephone service for patients to talk directly to a unit nurse. Thirdly, realistic pain expectations on the day of surgery and subsequently. Fourthly, any special arrangements required for children.

2.   *'must endeavour always to achieve, maintain and develop knowledge, skill and competence to respond to those needs and interests'.* This principle is more appropriately covered later in this chapter when updating is covered.

3.   *'must honestly acknowledge any limits of personal knowledge and skill and take steps to remedy any relevant deficits in order effectively and appropriately to meet the needs of patients and clients'.* The first part of this principle was covered earlier under the discussion of Clause 4 of the Code, but this sentence continues with mention of remedial action. Such action is up to the individual nurse in the first instance as part of her or his professional accountability, not her manager or her employer. Occasionally, nurses who are predominantly ward-based feel at a disadvantage because they do not go into theatre very often. It is up to these nurses to take the initiative and negotiate with their manager an updating period (the length being dependent on the number and type of procedures undertaken, in addition to the usual management considerations) either in the DSU theatres or, for more specialist aspects, main theatres. It is likely that there will be theatre nurses who wish to 'swap' to achieve updating in the ward area – admitting and discharging patients as well as pre- and post-operative nursing care.

4.   *'must ensure that any enlargement or adjustment of the scope of personal professional practice must be achieved without compromising or fragmenting existing aspects of professional practice and care and that the requirements of the Council's Code of Professional Conduct are satisfied throughout the whole area of practice'.* Perhaps one area where there is enlargement of a DSU nurse's knowledge and skill is for those who work predominantly in a scrubbed capacity in theatre. The number of trained staff required in theatre is three: two for the surgical care of the patient and one for the anaesthetic care. However, this can be compromised if the scrubbed nurse also has to act as the surgical assistant because the consultant fails to bring a junior along to help. Where does her priority lie – with her duty of care to the surgical patient,

for example, preventing diathermy injuries and maintaining correct 'counts', or with the consultant for whom she is performing the tasks of a houseman, for example, cleaning and draping and/or retracting instruments? As procedures become more complex, it will be essential for the nurse to make a choice – does she stay as the scrubbed nurse or does she become one of the new breed of surgical assistants with all the appropriate and necessary training for the role. (This role is mentioned later in this chapter when professional courses are considered.)

5.   *'must recognise and honour the direct or indirect personal accountability borne for all aspects of professional practice...'.* DSU nurses will come across many different patient scenarios when they perform pre-assessment interviews. During this process they must use their own personal judgement to analyse some delicate situations. Such situations may include patients who fall just outside the criteria for day surgery. For example, a patient may admit to drinking more than the accepted daily units of alcohol. However, in her or his patient education role, she or he discovers that this patient's wife has just been diagnosed with a terminal disease and his drinking is to relieve his stress. The DSU nurse now has a dilemma – does she or he state the patient is outside the criteria and transfer him to the in-patient list? Or does she appreciate the patient's social situation, noting the need for him to have surgery quickly so he can return to caring for his wife? If the latter course of action is chosen in negotiation with the patient, the DSU nurse should continue in her or his patient education role, emphasising the importance of a reduction in alcohol intake in the days prior to surgery to ensure a safer recovery from general anaesthesia.

6.   *'must, in serving the interests of patients and clients and the wider interests of society avoid any inappropriate delegation to others which compromises those interests'.* This returns us to the role of day surgery patient carers. If carers are not happy about taking responsibility for the patient if they appear, for example, to be in a lot of pain, then discussion should take place regarding the patient's admission to an in-patient bed. Failure to listen to their concerns means they reluctantly take the patient home. Once home, they can become more and more anxious. Anxiety displayed by the carer can be transferred to the patient, who should be resting and feeling generally supported. With the cutbacks and reorganisations across the community health

care sector, the carer's anxiety can be further heightened if they telephone the patient's GP and are put through to a locum service. The locum may not even be aware of the patient's admission for day surgery. Should this spiral go out of control, the patient could become a re-admission statistic.

In terms of numbers of patients being treated on a day basis, it is possible that carers will one day be patients themselves. They will either face this as a normal health care event or with trepidation because they have recollections of previous inappropriate actions. This is even more important in relation to children who, if they have a satisfactory day surgery 'journey' will not grow up in fear of another hospital encounter (which so many of us have had in the past).

Professional courses for qualified nurses and placement ideas for diploma students

Nurse education has seen numerous changes in the past five years, which has culminated in nurse education provision coming under the auspices of university faculties. This means that within a health sciences-related faculty, nurses will now be educated alongside phys-iotherapists, radiographers and pharmacologists, which can only give these professions a healthy awareness and respect for each other. The only group missing are the doctors, who remain with their traditional medical schools.

One of the difficulties for nurses in recent years has been in obtaining study leave, as increasing numbers of patients are treated and, simultaneously, nursing posts are being frozen. This has led to a move away from longer 6–12-month post-registration courses to more flexible day-release schemes. Such schemes have lent them-selves, in university terms, to the creation of whole or half modules of learning. The structure of a module relates to a given number of learning hours, which may be in the classroom with teacher contact, in related clinical practice, or in private study. The learning hours for a module comprise approximately 120–150 hours in total for 30 academic credits. University courses are generally offered at diploma, degree, masters and doctoral levels. Students must attain 120 credits at level II for a diploma course and 120 credits at level III for a degree course and so forth. Entrance into a particular course usually (but not always) means that the student has already achieved 120 credits at the previous level.

The nursing, midwifery and health visiting professions have their own new structure for professional and academic development. This structure includes the Framework for Continuing Professional Education and ENB Higher Award (ENB, 1990b). The Framework is based around 10 key characteristics (see Table 9.1) that describe the qualities of practitioners working with clients. Practitioners, in conjunction with service and educational managers, can negotiate a series of modules and register for the Higher Award to acquire the 10 key characteristics. The Higher Award is equivalent to a Bachelor (Honours) degree.

Table 9.1: The 10 key characteristics

1. Professional accountability and responsibility
2. Clinical expertise with a specific client group
3. Using research to plan, implement and evaluate strategies to improve care
4. Teamworking and building, multidisciplinary team leadership
5. Flexible and innovative approaches to care
6. Use of health promotion strategies
7. Facilitating and assessing development in others
8. Handling information and making informed clinical decisions
9. Setting standards and evaluating quality of care
10. Instigating, managing and evaluating clinical change

Reproduced with kind permission of the English National Board for Nursing, Midwifery and Health Visiting.

Practitioners are now eligible for accreditation of prior learning (APL) for certified courses, including ENB post-registration clinical courses undertaken within the past five years. This means they can achieve academic credit for coursework if it is deemed at the appropriate level and relates to the 10 key characteristics. Coursework not meeting these conditions can be supplemented by the practitioner, with tutorial support and then submitted to the APL faculty board for acceptance. This scheme prevents repetition of content material. Twinned with APL, is accreditation of prior experiential learning (APEL). If practitioners have undertaken courses in, for instance, counselling or business studies, they can prepare a portfolio of evidence indicating how the theory of the course has been applied to practice in their particular workplace to claim academic credit.

The *Day Surgery Task Force Report* (NHSME, 1993a) took the education and training of all personnel in this area very seriously, dedicating a whole section of their toolkit to the subject. For nurses, they recommend the formal teaching of an eclectic and holistic role with the generation of skills ranging from assessment to liaison upon discharge of the patient, in addition to the acute hospital skills in anaesthesia, theatre and recovery.

In the past five years, the ENB has approved two post-registration day surgery courses. The first of these, ENB A21 (Peri-operative and day care nursing practice), is known as the 'long' course, with participants completing 300 hours of theory and 600 hours of practice. This course contains four fundamental theoretical themes (see Table 9.2) which are developed throughout, plus specific themes, for example, history of day surgery; pre-assessment; American Society of Anesthesiologists (ASA) classification; considerations of different client groups undergoing day surgery; development and impact of minimal access techniques; pain management; concerns of carers and health economics (to name but a few). For the practice element of the course participants have to keep a reflective diary and a reading log indicating how they have met the course outcomes in conjunction with the 10 key characteristics. When participants have successfully completed the course, most educational institutions will award 60 level II credits.

Table 9.2: Fundemental theoretical themes for ENB A21

- Frameworks of nursing care
- Methods of enquiry
- Applied sciences
- Patient education and information-giving

One of the difficulties at the commencement of this course was the limited availability of experienced mentors to guide and support course members through their programme. This meant that a lot of the course tutor's time was spent with mentors and managers discussing the course programme and how the theory and practice elements linked together. The necessary course documentation was explained and details were worked out to facilitate moves within the course member's own DSU to achieve practice outcomes and, where necessary, to visit other units for specialist experiences. At the time, day surgery was a new specialty and the development of procedures and nursing care was changing rapidly. This put a lot of additional pressure on some key clinical staff but they rose to the challenge as they recognised the opportunities that were unfolding. These opportunities included a potential place on the course for themselves, enhanced patient care and improved standards throughout the unit.

The second course, N33 (Peri-operative and day care nursing practice for experienced day surgery nurses), known as the 'short' course, comprises 10 study days and enables practitioners to update and develop their knowledge and skills in this specialist area of nursing. (Readers wishing to find out where either course is run are advised to contact the ENB direct.)

There are other clinical courses available for nurses who wish to specialise in a specific area within the day surgery setting:

- ENB 176 (Operating department nursing);
- ENB 182 (Anaesthetic nursing);
- ENB 183 (Operating department and anaesthetic nursing);
- ENB 346 (Ophthalmic nursing).

As mentioned earlier, nearly all clinical courses are made up of half or whole modules and if participants have already embarked on ENB A21 they may wish to choose just a single module from, say, three, which make up the total for the course. This will obviously depend on how the course has been designed. For example, in the author's previous faculty ENB 346 comprised two half modules and one whole module. In conjunction with educational and service managers, it may only be deemed appropriate for a course participant to pursue the second half module because it pertains to acute ophthalmic practice, which is the care this group of patients most often seeks in day surgery.

Nurses specialising in the theatre area of day surgery may be interested in a newly developed ENB short course, N77 (Nurse as assistant to the surgeon). With the reduction in junior doctors' hours, some nurses may wish to respond to this innovative course within the UKCC *Scope of Professional Practice* (UKCC, 1992b). But are nurses who take on this expanded role leaving a void in the theatre caring role? Is quality care allowing untrained personnel (health care assistants) to fill this void? Perhaps in the day surgery environment where there is a high proportion of trained staff this will not happen and opportunities will present where nurse surgical assistants can really develop. Health care assistants do have a role in day surgery but the emphasis must be upon care assessed, planned, delivered and evaluated by registered nurses to this potentially vulnerable group of clients who receive surgery within an eight-hour period (home to home).

And what of our community colleagues? As increasing numbers of day patients are treated, invariably some have to be followed up in the community. The roles and workload of community nurses are changing in a similar way to those of nurses in the acute sector, so they too need updating. Modules can be designed and implemented for community staff to critically review patient preparation for surgery, for example, pre-assessment whether undertaken in the primary care or acute setting; the impact that new technology such as laser, endoscopy and microwave has on patient treatments; and lastly, evaluation of discharge and follow-up protocols for patients and carers returning home.

The Royal College of Surgeons (1992) recommended that 50 per cent of elective surgery is performed on a day case basis by the end of the millenium. If this target is achieved, then it seems wholly inappropriate for participants on the diploma education programme leading to registration, to spend just two days in the day surgery setting. These will be our nurses of the future so it is important for them to understand and appreciate the benefits of day surgery for both patients and the health service. And it is hoped that this will encourage them to look forward to building upon its current success.

Within education circles, there is some debate as to whether the day surgery allocation falls into the community or the acute setting. Some would say it fits into both. To enable a diploma student to focus on the continuous (if short-term) care of a patient undergoing day surgery she or he should be able to see how the patient is initially referred or fast-tracked for treatment. She or he should then be able to understand and undertake supervised care in the acute setting and, finally, follow the patient back into the community.

With creative planning, it should be possible to arrange a community link in the common foundation programme (CFP – the first 18 months of the programme), for example, accompanying a district nurse when she is undertaking a pre-assessment of the home circumstances if the DSU has requested one; then an acute placement in the branch programme (the final 18 months of the programme). In the branch programme diploma students have the ideal opportunity in a day surgery setting to consolidate a number of concepts acquired in the CFP, for example, patient assessment techniques and all the associated interpersonal and communication skills; anatomy and physiology; care of the unconscious patient and discharge planning.

To set the scene, diploma students need a preparation day in the university. Typical content for such a study day could include:

- history of day surgery;
- procedures that can be performed;
- assessment and planning of care using a nursing model, e.g. Orem;

- importance of good communication – verbal and written;
- multifaceted role of the nurse in day surgery.

This content should be supplemented with a thorough reading list so that diploma students are well armed with theoretical knowledge when they arrive for their clinical placement. Here, under the supervision of a mentor they can participate in the requisite day surgery nursing care, and specifically planned practice outcomes will ensure this is achieved.

Until the 1990s, clinical updating tended to be organised either by enthusiatic managers or motivated individual practitioners. Such managers encourage weekly teaching sessions; support the formation and ongoing work of quality circles; or facilitate visits to other DSUs for their own staff and allow visits to their unit by external staff. As well as attending recognised courses, individual nurses may supplement their knowledge through reading appropriate day surgery literature and share this new information with peers, possibly in the form of a learning resource. Additionally, they may attend specialist day surgery conferences in their own time and/or at their own expense.

A recent concept that aims to enhance updating is clinical supervision. The NHS Management Executive states that 'clinical supervision is a term used to describe a formal process of professional support and learning which enables individual practitioners to develop knowledge and competence, assume responsibility for their own practice and enhance consumer protection and the safety of care in complex clinical situations' (NHSME, 1993b, p. 15). According to Kohner (1994) a number of nursing development units (NDU) have quickly adopted this concept, tailoring different systems of clinical supervision to their own particular needs. In line with so many ideas in nursing, systems of clinical supervision should not be 'set in stone', they need to be carefully planned, implemented, monitored and evaluated. For this to work requires the commitment of all staff at all levels. As it is a relatively new concept, many managers are initiating clinical supervision systems by acting as supervisors for their staff, but in NDUs where clinical supervision has become well established, supervisees have chosen their own supervisors, who may well be peers. The functions of clinical supervision are (in a nutshell) to improve the quality of patient care and to acknowledge the value of staff who work in areas of high patient turnover, such as DSUs. Kohner (1994) continued by exploring five case studies of NDUs utilising clinical supervision and some of the main elements are drawn out below:

- it provides support in the development of practitioners' practice;
- it expands on the *Scope of Professional Practice*;
- it uses reflection to increase self-awareness, assertiveness and confidence;
- it facilitates the link between theory and practice through the emphasis on research;
- it encourages broad thinking, which increases the options available to practitioners;
- clinical supervision is a two-way formal process that is either documented or taped. Frequently, contracts are utilised after discussion of the ground rules concerning the frequency and timing of sessions, otherwise there can be a tendency for 'grousing sessions' to occur.

So, what could clinical supervision have to offer day surgery nurses? It should enable them to feel supported, which can be a difficult concept to achieve when the speed and pressure of work can be demanding. If each and every nurse knows that they will receive clinical supervision then they will more readily cover for one another. It encourages personal and professional growth, as staff have got to know that someone is aware of the demands of their home life and how this interfaces with maintaining their professional development. There is a greater sense of commitment if all members of the day surgery nursing team are given equity in the clinical supervision process. This, in turn will build staff confidence and improve teamwork.

Does clinical supervision have a down-side? According to Fox (1994) it does. The nursing workforce has now become flexible, with nurses working full-time, part-time and on the 'bank' in the majority of DSUs. This could mean a lot of repetition in terms of introducing a system of clinical supervision. Trained nurses are also now in the minority, with more care duties resting with health care assistants and informal carers. These personnel require general supervision, which erodes time available for clinical supervision. Perhaps this latter point could be used to make a claim for additional trained nursing staff in DSUs.

'Post-Registration Education and Practice (PREP) is the term used to describe the UKCC's requirements for education and practice following registration' (UKCC, 1995, fact sheet 1). The purpose of PREP is to improve standards of patient care and act as a public check that a nurse has the qualifications to provide safe care.

Registered nurses who renew their registration after 1 April 1995 will be informed of their PREP requirements to be met before they re-register again in three years' time. There are four key elements to maintain registration. Firstly, notification to practise will check personal data and will also request further information about a practitioner's specific area of practice, their employer and how many hours the practitioner intends to work. Secondly, the undertaking of a minimum of five study days. This point is examined in more detail below. Thirdly, to maintain a personal professional portfolio (PPP). This is an account of a practitioner's clinical and educational development and how this was achieved. Fourthly, to undertake a Return to Practice programme (statutory from 1 April 2000) if a nurse has been out of practice for five years or more.

Returning to the minimum of five study days, the UKCC has created five broad categories to assist practitioners planning:

- patient, client and colleague support;
- care enhancement;
- practice development;
- reducing risk;
- educational development (UKCC, 1995, fact sheet 3).

Practitioners are advised to plan their development carefully – setting objectives, creating and carrying out an action plan and, finally, evaluating learning. Accurate record-keeping is advocated, linking in with the PPP accounting for study time and learning outcomes. How can day surgery nurses use the five broad categories?

Patient, client and colleague support

The previous section in this chapter looked at clinical supervision and it may be feasible for a group of day surgery nurses to undertake a literature search related to this topic and initiate a pilot scheme within their unit. It may also be pertinent to establish a support group for day surgery carers, or a liaison group between nurses in a DSU and local GP practice nurses to discuss areas of common concern.

Care enhancement

Care enhancement is a very topical area in day surgery as more and more procedures and techniques are being carried out in DSUs. This could be an opportunity for nurses not familiar with endoscopic or minimally invasive techniques to enhance their knowledge and practice. Even nurses who work predominantly in the ward will find it beneficial to go into theatre and observe such procedures. It will give them a better insight into what happens to the patient under sedation or anaesthesia and, additionally, it provides them with accurate (because it is first-hand) information should patients or carers ask them questions.

Practice development

This is an important learning opportunity for day surgery nurses. However good a DSU is, there is always room for improvement. Nurses should negotiate with managers to visit other units that may have specific expertise, for example, a paediatric DSU, a hospital hotel, or a cardiac day unit. A clinical visit not only enables nurses to fulfil specific objectives, but broadens learning by looking at the geographical layout of a unit, observing the staffing levels and mix, talking to the staff – medical, nursing and ancillary – and communicating with the patients. All these aspects can be very enlightening.

Reducing risk

An example for completing this category could be observing and reviewing information sheets for day surgery patients. There is a tendency to understate the obvious. Patients are always told prior to a general anaesthetic to have nothing to eat or drink, but they are rarely told why. Patient compliance with care is better if they understand the rationale for what they have been requested to do, or not do. Similarly, with post-operative information sheets, self-care can be enhanced if rationales follow required actions, for example, care following hand surgery. The action would be to keep the hand elevated, and the associated rationale would be because this will help to reduce swelling and make the hand more comfortable.

Educational development

When nurses see the word 'research' they tend to panic, but it should not be beyond any trained nurse to undertake a small-scale piece of research. The author has been involved with a DSU where the nurses have looked at some of the following issues: why gynaecological patients get more pain than other client groups; do carers understand their role?; and patients' perceptions of day surgery. The key to research is to stay with a problem that intrigues you and endeavour to look for an answer. Where possible, gain the support of the unit manager and peers, all of whom can be influential motivating forces. Finally, follow the steps of the research process:

- undertake a literature review;
- plan the study;
- undertake a pilot study;
- collect the main study data;
- interpret the results;
- draw conclusions;
- share the completed study with colleagues.

Details for each of these points may be obtained from any standard text on nursing research.

PREP appears to be daunting in many respects, but in a positive light, it is striving to improve practitioners' development and ultimately the care given to day surgery patients. Challenging times are ahead for us all.

At various points in this chapter, it has been suggested that staff in the DSU should be allowed to move to all areas within the unit and observe and participate in patient care in some capacity. The most crucial time for this to occur is when new staff join a DSU and need an induction programme. Sutherland (1994) described the programme that his unit developed for a ward nurse. The programme was based on an initial four-week period and included a general introduction, unit documentation, theatre routines, anaesthetic and recovery routines, and practice within the ward. However, the programme is ongoing for a period extending over 12 months, with similar programmes set for nurses specialising in theatres, anaesthetics or recovery. He suggested programmes should be made available for clerical and ancillary staff too. On talking to day surgery nurses, it would appear that one week in each of the areas is too short. Depending on the number of different medical and surgical specialties and the specialist client groups the DSU caters for, the process of learning could take up to one month in each of the areas.

The future

Nurses working in DSUs have a very demanding and responsible role within the acute health care sector, where they work from 07.30 am to 7.30 pm Monday to Friday (however, this is likely to change in response to consumer demand). Although Treloar (1989) argues that these hours are very appealing as they offer no night or weekend duties and offer flexibility to part-time staff, the hours still create problems. Not least for the education and training of personnel.

What are the most appropriate times for study release? Who pays for study? The author, working in a provider service, when endeavoured to offer study flexibly, in the evening or at weekends.

Theoretically, this is sound, but practically, it is not feasible for day surgery nurses who have no energy left at the end of the day for study, and would see education at the weekend as an infringement of their private and recreational time. This is without the added problem of travelling. Education provision is now more centralised so staff are having to travel greater distances to attend courses.

One answer, but not the complete answer, is the introduction of day surgery distance learning materials. Distance learning is a highly flexible mode of study but it does not suit everyone. Principally, it is guided, independent study, but participants should be offered periodic group tutorials to lend support. Lack of support is one of the main reasons why distance learning fails because participants can feel so isolated in their learning.

Post-registration courses for trained nurses have already been mentioned, but one of the advantages of nurse education moving into universities has to be the higher academic programmes that can be developed. It is to be hoped that within the next five years, degrees and masters programmes will be available for day surgery nurses to tap into. Such programmes will enable topics to be explored in real depth, for instance, do surgical patients really choose day case treatment?; is there a need for community nurse attachment to DSUs to target the follow-up of specific patients? These programmes can only promote excellence in practice, further more research opportunities and enhance day surgery patient care.

An area of concern is that, in some instances, day surgery is losing its specialist identity. A growing number of managers appear to want to use day surgery as an extension of the main operating department. This was echoed to some extent by the Director of the National Association of Community Health Councils at the 1995 BADS conference when he commented 'My concern is that the managerial drive to reduce or shift costs will lead to unacceptable pressure on practitioners to perform day surgery in inappropriate cases...'.

In some areas staff are being told they have to rotate through the main operating department for extended periods. In theory this is sound, because practice development can be improved, but alarm bells ring when general theatre nurses are in short supply and day surgery nurses are possibly being used to make up the shortfall. It has also been noticed that staff are being encouraged to attend theatre and anaesthetic courses in preference to day surgery courses. While specialist day surgery courses facilitate competency in theatre and anaesthetics, by virtue of their length, these courses cannot go into the same depth as the theatre and anaesthetic courses. Day surgery courses offer a much broader base exploring issues outside the acute surgical phase – does the patient understand what day surgery is?; are the patient and carer happy to participate in self-care?; are there specific problems for elderly patients undergoing day surgery?; what complications can arise when the patient returns home? These issues would not be addressed in either a theatre or anaesthetic course. A possible way of combining all areas of knowledge and skills could be a diploma/degree in day surgery with a set number of compulsory modules, and a choice of other modules from a menu (see Table 9.3).

Table 9.3: Menu of modules for inclusion in a diploma/degree in day surgery

Compulsory modules	Selection menu of modules
Fundamentals of day surgery care	Care of the paediatric day surgery patient
Anaesthetic patient care	Care of the patient undergoing endoscopy
Theatre patient care	Advanced day surgery practice
Recovery patient care	Day surgery patients in the community
	Day surgery management
	Day surgery budgeting
	Research in day surgery

Clinical competencies have evolved for day surgery practice in conjunction with post-registration courses (Hodge, 1994), but why have these competencies not been published widely for comment by day surgery practitioners? Surely such competencies should be available to all DSUs (especially those at the bottom of the learning curve) and not reserved solely for those fortunate enough to attend courses. Maybe this would bring out into the open the whole issue of multi-skilling in day surgery and the practices which nurses must, should and could be performing. The annual autumn Royal College of Nursing conference on day surgery could be dedicated to discussion on this one issue alone.

A development that DSUs could examine is that of the post of lecturer-practitioner (LP). This is a joint appointee paid for and managed by education and service managers, each with their own expectations of what the post entails. The reason for the creation of the LP post was, and remains, to bridge the theory/practice divide in nursing. The 'lecturer' aspect for the postholder means having a teaching commitment in an academic institution. The 'practitioner' aspect expects a professional with a patient caseload and, additionally,

responsibility for diploma students' achievement of clinical competencies, plus the continuing education of all other unit staff. The
demands and skills for each aspect are very different, which, according to Wright (1988), inevitably leads to conflict and overload. The
role requires adequate support, time and resources for it to be
successful. This is without the further complication of service and
education contractual arrangements when trusts are financially
independent and health care education has moved into academic
institutions.

What could such a post offer day surgery staff? Someone who is
skilled in day surgery practice and management; someone who can
provide a conducive learning environment and create learning
resources for staff; someone who can initiate and promote research
within the day surgery setting. Such a person could also have the
effect of raising morale and motivating staff.

BADS

This multidisciplinary day surgery association has been established
for some years now and has incorporated into its aims 'to promote
education and research in the field of day surgery'. But as yet there is
no educational subcommittee actively to further these aims. All
development is becoming more academically demanding whether
one is a nurse, doctor or ancillary grade, and sound, up-to-date
support must be co-ordinated and available to enable professionals
to go forward. Such a subcommittee is urgently needed. There is an
equally urgent need for some kind of centralised resource facility.
The *Journal of One Day Surgery* provides abstracts of recently published
books and articles, but the small number summarised each quarter
does not reflect the now abundant literature on day surgery. There is
also the problem of the heavy medical bias of most of these publications. Perhaps the educational subcommittee could run 'how to get
material published' seminars for nurses and other interested parties,
to redress this balance. A resource centre could hold a stock of videos
and other teaching aids which could be loaned to universities or
DSUs for a modest charge. Professional life is tough and any assistance for personnel will surely lighten their load.

Medical staff

This final section considers some of the issues surrounding the
training of our medical colleagues. The DSU is considered to be the
domain of the consultants, who are able to perform efficiently and
effectively. They are experienced and can anticipate potential

complications. This results in a first-class service facilitating surgery in a day and a trouble-free recovery upon the patient's return home. But, how do junior doctors gain the necessary knowledge and experience in day surgery?

Some years ago the answer was that they could go to main theatres, where similar procedures were performed. However, surgical treatment delivery has moved on and the majority of minor surgery is now performed in DSUs. Some senior doctors do permit junior doctors to perform day surgery, which has advantages and disadvantages. The advantages tend to benefit the junior doctor. If the idea is to train the consultants of the future then it is important for them to be exposed to day surgery and to participate in it. The patients of the future will expect their doctors to have been appropriately trained in this growing area. The disadvantages affect the current patients, who will spend longer under anaesthesia and could suffer more tissue handling as anatomy is recognised and operation techniques are perfected. This could mean a patient's recovery is impeded while the increased amount of anaesthetic is broken down and excreted from the body, and possibly more bruising and pain in the area surrounding the wound.

So, what is the answer? Ideally, well equipped and properly resourced day surgery training centres would be the solution (but questionably feasible in a cash-strapped NHS). Computer software could be available to revise and update junior doctors' knowledge of anatomy and physiology. Surgical instrumentation and suture materials must be available for them to handle and manipulate so they do not slow down surgery unnecessarily. Use should be made of the latest technology, for example, closed circuit television with a two-way communication link into theatre areas so junior doctors could have direct observation of surgical procedures and dialogue with the operator. Carefully designed and thorough learning programmes with specific learning outcomes will enable medical students/junior doctors to access all the aforementioned resources as well as undertake supervised clinical teaching with day surgery patients. With the ethos of multidisciplinary approaches to day surgery, it is anticipated all other health care staff would have access to these learning resources too.

References

Bloom BS (Ed) (1956) Taxonomy of Educational Objectives. London: Longman.

English National Board (1990a) Regulations and Guidelines for the Approval of Institutions and Courses. London: ENB.

English National Board (1990b) A New Structure for Professional Development. The Framework for Continuing Professional Education and the ENB Higher Award for Nurses, Midwives and Health Visitors. London: ENB.

Fox J (1994) Editorial. Clinical supervision: a real aspiration? British Journal of Nursing (16): 805.

Gale L, Pol G (1977) Determining required competence: a need assessment methodology and computer programme. Educational Technology 17: 24–28.

Green D (1995) Patient assessment in day surgery. British Journal of Theatre Nursing 5(1): 10–12.

Hill G, Roberts G (1992) Risk management in day unit surgery. Journal of One Day Surgery 2(1): 8–9.

Hodge D (1994) Introduction to day surgery. Surgical Nurse 7(2): 12–16.

Kalideen D (1991) The case for preoperative visiting. British Journal of Theatre Nursing 1(5): 19–22.

Kenworthy N (1995) Editorial. Multi-skilling. Professional Update 3(5): 33.

Kohner N (1994) Clinical Supervision in Practice. London: Kings Fund Centre.

NHS Management Executive (1993a) Day Surgery. Report by the Day Surgery Task Force. London: HMSO.

NHS Management Executive (1993b) A Vision for the Future. The Nursing, Midwifery and Health Visiting Contribution to Health and Health Care. London: HMSO.

Penn S (1990) Day surgery. British Journal of Theatre Nursing 27(10): 3–4.

Reid T (1995) Taken to task. Nursing Times 91(21): 18.

Roy S (1996) Risk management. Nursing Standard 10(18): 51–54.

Royal College of Surgeons of England (1992) Commission on the Provision of Surgical Services. Report of the Working Party on Guidelines for Day Case Surgery. London: RCS.

Sutherland R (1994) Is this the way forward? British Journal of Theatre Nursing 4(1): 12–13.

Taylor M (1993) Universal Precautions in the operating department. British Journal of Theatre Nursing 2(10): 4–7.

Treloar E (1989) Establishing a day care unit (b) in private practice. In Bradshaw E, Davenport H (Eds), Day Care. Surgery, Anaesthesia and Management. London: Edward Arnold.

United Kingdom Central Council (1992a) The Code of Professional Conduct, 3rd edn. London: UKCC.

United Kingdom Central Council (1992b) The Scope of Professional Practice. London: UKCC.

United Kingdom Central Council (1993) Standards for Records and Record Keeping. London: UKCC.

United Kingdom Central Council (1995) PREP and You. London: UKCC.

Wright S (1988) Joint appointments: handle with care. Nursing Times 84(1): 32–33.

Index

accreditation of prior experiential
learning (APEL) 189
accreditation of prior learning (APL)
189
acetylcholine 52, 53, 54
adenoidectomy 89, 90, 140
admission to hospital 12, 161, 170
overnight 14, 20, 57, 58, 65–6, 167,
174
unplanned 102, 104, 121
adolescents 135, 136, 137
adrenalin 44, 47, 48, 58, 69, 90
age 17, 19, 21, 25–6
care of elderly patients 118–19, 124
agency nurses 159
airways 106–8
anaesthesia 42, 45, 55
children 142, 151, 152
pre-assessment 18, 20
recovery 97, 99, 105, 106–8
alarms 98, 180
alcohol 24, 100, 187
alfentanil 50, 103, 104
allergies 20, 42, 74, 106
American Society of Anesthesiologists
Classification 12, 13, 17, 43, 190
AMETOP 45
amputation of digits 2, 58, 87, 140
anaesthesia and anaesthetics 38–64,
110, 142–3
adverse effects 104
anxiety 22, 32, 39, 42, 44, 61

children 45–7, 49, 61, 136, 140–3,
145, 147, 152
complications 38, 41–2, 56–7
discharge 42, 62, 120–3
drugs commonly used 45–55
DSU design 166, 168, 169–70
history 3, 5, 6, 8
induction 6, 22, 32, 38–9, 42–50,
103
induction agents 18, 43, 44, 45–6,
47–9, 56, 61–2
maintenance 38–9, 42, 45–6, 47,
62, 103
non-nursing staff 160
nursing care 38–41
pre-assessment 14, 16–21, 23, 30,
32–4, 39–44, 54, 62
premedication 44–5
recovery 41–3, 45–6, 48–9, 51, 62,
96, 98–100, 103–5, 107–9
reversal 39, 45, 50, 52, 56, 108
selection 11, 13, 43
theatre 61, 67, 68, 73–4, 76, 77
training 41–2, 178–9, 182, 185–6,
190, 196–9, 201
see also general anaesthetic;
local anaesthetic
anaesthetic assistants 40, 42, 157, 160
anaesthetic nurses 39–42, 45, 53, 62,
104, 160
epidural 60
training 191